DISCARD

ENCYCLOPEDIA OF
FAMILY HEALTH

--- THIRD EDITION ---

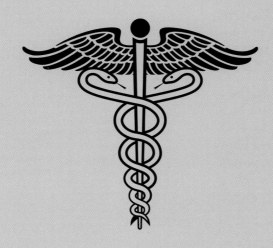

CONSULTANTS

David B. Jacoby, M.D.
Johns Hopkins School of Medicine

Robert M. Youngson, M.D.
Royal Society of Medicine

VOLUME 16

TAI CHI — TYPHUS

MARSHALL CAVENDISH
New York · London · Singapore

MEDICAL CONSULTANTS

Second Edition
David B. Jacoby, M.D.
Johns Hopkins School of Medicine
Associate Professor of Pulmonary and Critical
   Care Medicine

Third Edition
Robert M. Youngson, M.D.
Fellow of the Royal Society of Medicine
Officer of the Order of St John of Jerusalem
Diploma in Tropical Medicine and Hygiene
Fellow of the Royal College of Ophthalmologists

CONTRIBUTORS TO THIRD EDITION

David Arnot	Tom Jackson
Deborah Evans	Nathan Lepora
Leon Gray	Fiona Plowman
Joanna Griffin	Alison Tarrant
Tim Harris	Aruna Vasudevan
John Jackson	

Picture Credits
(b – bottom; t – top; r – right; l – left; c – center)

Cover: Digital Vision: c; Dynamic Graphics: John Foxx & Images 4
Communication b/l, b/r; PhotoDisc: Don Farrall b/c, Keith Brofsky t/r.

Alan Hutchinson Library: 2224, 2280t, 2290, 2297; All-Sport: 2187l; Ann Kelley:
2185; Ann Ronan Picture Library: 2255; ARS: Keith Weller 2249; Aspect Picture
Library: 2283; Biophoto Associates: 2173t, 2187r, 2198b, 2218, 2222, 2289all;
Bruce Coleman Ltd: 2184b, WWF/Eugen Schuhmacher 2184t; C James Webb:
2276, 2279l, 2281b/r, 2282l, 2298t/r, 2298b, 2300r; Charles Day: 2175r,
2177t/l; Colorific: Diane Wayman 2173b, Linda Bartlett 2188; Corbis: Chuck
Savage 2230b, Dann Tardif/LWA 2190, 2228, Ed Young 2263, Gabe Palmer
2225l, James L Amos 2265, Jim Cummins 2186, Joe McDonald 2301b, Jose Luis
Pelaez Inc 2206r, Larry Williams 2243, Lester V Bergman 2262b, Michael Keller
2260, Michael Prince 2279r, Neil Beckerman 2172, Nik Wheeler 2166, 2168l,
2206l, Paul Barton 2231r, 2168r, Peter Turnley 2267, Rob Lewine 2262t, Ronnie
Kaufman 2234b, Stephen Welstead/LWA 2171r, Steve Prezant 2231l, Tom
Stewart 2278, Wally McNamee 2266t, Warren Morgan 2268; Corbis Royalty
Free: 2269, 2299; Digital Vision: 2245; Dynamic Graphics: John Foxx & Images
4 Communication 2221, 2236, 2241r; Getty Images: 2182, 2193r, 2207,
2277b, 2284b/r, Elyse Lewin 2215b; Graham Strong: 2281t; Imagingbody.com:
2174, 2194; John Kevern: 2170; John Watney: 2237r; Ken Moreman: 2225c,
2287; London Scientific Fotos: 2247, 2193l; National Medical Slide Bank: 2219,
2237l; Oliver Hatch: 2256; Papilio: Jamie Harron 2300l; PHIL: Dr Thomas F
Sellers 2277t; PhotoDisc: Doug Menuez 2241l, Keith Brofsky 2175l, Russell Illig
2181, Suza Scalora 2239, 2242t; Photos.com: 2205, 2257, 2261, 2273; Rex
Features: 2210l, 24/7, AGB Photo Library 2242b, Alexander Caminada 2238,
Erik Pendzich 2189, Henryk T Kaiser 2234t, Ian Turner Worldwide 2202, Karl
Schoendorfer 2281b/l, M Towski/DMI 2244, Phanie Agency 2258, 2259, Sipa
Press 2264, Susa/Fotex 2274, TDY 2230t, Voisin/Phanie 2177b/l, 2179; Robert
Harding: 2195, 2301t; Roger Payling: 2210r, 2213; Ron Sutherland: 2248; Sally
& Richard Greenhill: 2197; Science Photo Library: 2196, Alex Bartel 2216,
BSIP/Laurent H Americain 2291, David Montrose 2208, Dr P Marazzi 2220, John
Greim 2214, Larry Mulvehill 2253, Richard T Nowitz 2177b/r; Steve
Bielschowsky: 2212all, 2232; Shout Pictures: 2275, 2293, 2294; Topham
Picturepoint: Joe Carini/The Image Works 2165, Karen Preuss/ The Image Works
2171l, Larry Mulvehill/The Image Works 2199, The Image Works 2209; US
Department of Defense: 2227; USDA/NRCS: Charlie Rahm 2198t; Vision
International: CNRI 2215t, 2292all, Errath/Explorer 2280b, Hervy/Explorer
2284t, Paolo Koch 2183, Veron/Explorer 2284b/l; Wellcome Photo Library:
2200, 2252, 2254; Zefa: 2229, 2270, 2271.

Marshall Cavendish
99 White Plains Road
Tarrytown, NY 10591-9001

www.marshallcavendish.com

© 2005, 1998, 1991 Marshall Cavendish Corporation

Library of Congress Cataloging-in-Publication Data

Encyclopedia of family health / David B. Jacoby, Robert M. Youngson.--
3rd ed.
      p. cm.
Includes bibliographical references and index.
   ISBN 0-7614-7486-2 (set)
   ISBN 0-7614-7502-8 (vol 16)
1. Medicine, Popular--Encyclopedias. 2. Health--Encyclopedias. 1. Jacoby, David
B. II. Youngson, R. M. III. Marshall Cavendish Corporation. IV. Title
RC81.A2E5 2004
610'.3--dc22   2003065554

Printed in China
08 07 06 05 04 5 4 3 2 1

Marshall Cavendish

Editor: Joyce Tavolacci
Editorial Director: Paul Bernabeo
Production Manager: Alan Tsai

The Brown Reference Group

Project Editor: Anne Hildyard
Editors: Jane Lanigan, Sally McFall
Designers: Jeni Child, Reg Cox, Karen Frazer
Picture Researcher: Clare Newman
Indexer: Kay Ollerenshaw
Illustrations: Samantha J. Elmhurst
Managing Editor: Tim Cooke
Art Director: Dave Goodman

CONTENTS

KEY TO COLOR CODING OF ARTICLES

- HUMAN BODY
- DISEASES AND OTHER DISORDERS
- TREATMENTS AND CURES
- PREVENTION AND DIAGNOSIS OF DISEASE
- HUMAN BEHAVIOR

Tai chi

Questions and Answers

How does slow movement in tai chi help to maintain the physique?

The aim of tai chi, which is a series of slow body movements, is to relax the body and the mind so that the person is prepared for an effective defense against illness and psychological disorders. Physical benefits that can be derived from tai chi are greater flexibility, improved circulation, better balance, and also an enhanced sense of well-being.

Is tai chi similar to yoga?

Only in the sense that it relaxes both the body and the mind. The main physical activity of tai chi is different from yoga in that it is carried out standing up, using balletlike movements of the legs and the arms. Yoga is a system of exercises, postures, meditation, breathing, and relaxation, which is performed standing up, in a sitting position, or lying down. The aim is similar; to achieve a balance of body and mind.

Do you need to be strong to practice tai chi?

Not necessarily. Physical strength is not needed for the fluid movements. A degree of strength is required, since you have to hold a position before moving with ease to the next one. What is necessary, however, is to have the capacity for concentration.

Can anybody practice tai chi?

Yes. Age and sex are not barriers. Many people take it up for the first time in their middle or later years in order to try to find peace of mind and to restore a balance in their working and private lives. You can practice tai chi anywhere—in your living room, the garden, or even the office.

Tai chi is a Chinese martial art that was developed several hundred years ago. It is valued for improving fitness, health, and longevity, and is now one of the most popular ways to exercise both the body and the mind.

The Chinese call this ancient martial art tàijíquán, but Westerners refer to it colloquially as tai chi chuan or tai chi. Over 10 million people carry out this elegant form of exercise every day in China, and its popularity has spread from Asia during the past 30 years to countries such as Japan, Australia, the United States, Canada, and many European countries.

The philosophy of tai chi

Tai chi promotes complete bodily and mental relaxation. There are five main styles, each of them based on similar principles. The name tai chi chuan means "supreme ultimate fist," and is taken for the concept and philosophy of tai chi, which is symbolized in the ancient symbols of yin and yang—the inviolable duality. The light and the dark of the yin-yang symbol represent the two central forces in the universe around us. The two symbols are linked by a smaller circle within the center of each, representing its opposite.

The movements in tai chi are characterized by a yielding element, and by a continuous flow of energy. It is a play of opposites. Every movement is circular and as a result of each movement, the opposite is revealed. The opposites are: sinking followed by rising up; pulling back, then reaching out; and moving left in order to swing right.

The form

Solo practice, known as the form, is a precisely choreographed sequence of movements lasting for anything between five and 60 minutes, depending on which version or style is practiced. Every movement is carried out in slow motion and is accompanied by regular breathing.

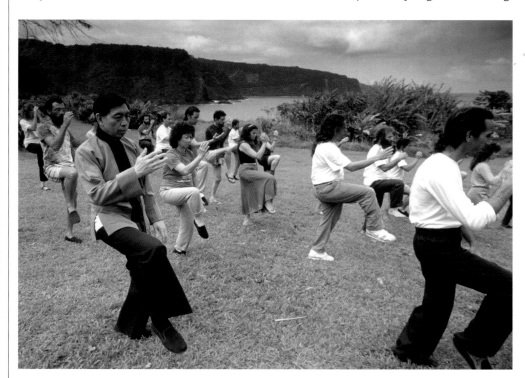

▲ *People practice tai chi in a park in Maui, Hawaii. Its popularity has spread from China to the rest of the world, and it is now practiced in many Western countries.*

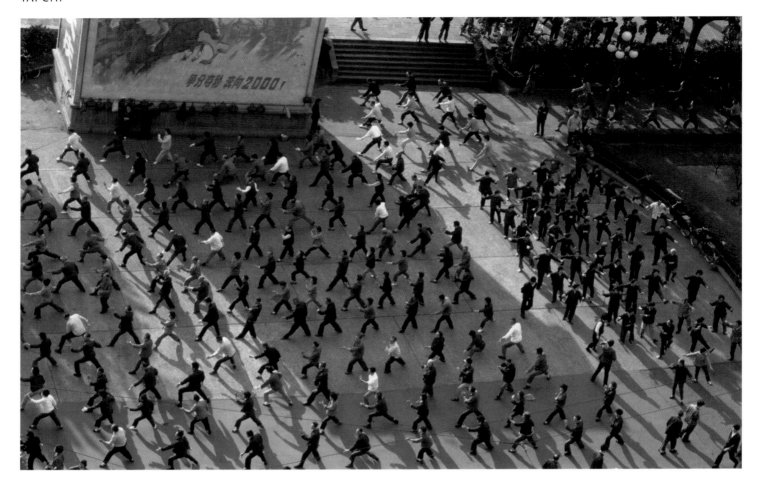

▲ *Tai chi can be practiced in almost any environment, either by one person or in a group. In China it is common for large groups of people to gather for daily practice.*

Movements are coordinated with the breathing so that the breath and body are in harmony.

The aim of serious practitioners—or players, as they are referred to in China—is to harmonize the various parts of the body, the emotions, and the spirit, while at the same time becoming conscious of states that are conflicting with each other such as tension and relaxation, which exist in the body and the mind.

Since tai chi is a martial art, practice can also include exercising with weapons, self-defense stances, and perhaps contact sparring. It can also involve standing in a particular posture for as little as a few minutes or as long as an hour. This discipline creates a state of spiritual peace, develops inner strength, and centers the body.

Among the guiding principles that underlie the concept of tai chi are relaxation, coordination, slow and continuous movement, cultivation of a calm psychological state and a clear spirit, and finding the center of energy that each of us has, or sinking as it is called in this form of martial art. Balance has to be achieved because some of the stances are in preparation for defending oneself, and to be unbalanced would be to be vulnerable.

Relaxation

Relaxation is the most important aim of tai chi. It is achieved by a range of warmup exercises that extend the arms, legs, and torso as well as loosen the joints. Another reason why is it essential for the body to be relaxed is so that the back and shoulders, the arms and legs, and the hips are all correctly aligned. Correct alignment allows ease of movement into different postures.

Coordination

Every movement of the sequence should be coordinated carefully so that the whole body is connected. Each movement involves concentrating on encouraging energy to flow up through the legs, hips, back, and shoulders, and out into the air through the arms and hands. Although the energy cannot be seen, practitioners of tai chi claim that they can feel it around them.

Slow and continuous movement

Once the movement has started, the aim is to keep it a continuous one, with no pausing or stopping in the sequence. Although the speed of the movement can vary depending on the style or physical limitations of an individual, there must not be even the slightest pause between movements.

Calm state and clear spirit

The process of achieving calmness and a clear spirit should be sought from the first day someone begins to study tai chi.

A student will be taught that the daily practice of the art helps to build up a sense of calm. This sense of calmness when someone is practicing tai chi also promotes a sense of well-being in all other areas of the practitioner's life.

Ten main points of Yang Ching-Pu (grandson of the founder of the Yang school)

1. Suspend the head from above and keep it up straight. This will enable your inner strength to reach the crown and your spirit will soar free. Keep your neck relaxed—a stiff neck becomes an obstacle to achieving this.

2. Depress the chest and raise the upper back. This way, you can sink the energy into your "tan-tien" and this, in turn, enables you to bring inner strength to your vertebrae.

3. Loosen the waist, a key point of the body. Loosening your waist allows you to anchor your feet and make the body secure.

4. Distinguish between solidness and emptiness. Once you have learned this, through moving weight from the left leg to the right and back again, your movements will be light-footed.

5. Droop the shoulders and sink the elbows. Loosening the shoulder joints allows energy to flow freely.

6. Apply will and not force. Completely relax the body while practicing tai chi. Awkward tensions in the body hinder the flow of energy.

7. Coordinate upper and lower body movements. Inner strength is centered in the feet, developed in the thighs, controlled by the waist, and expressed through the fingers.

8. Unify internal and external movements. Working on the theory that the spirit is the master and the body is the servant, the individual practitioner must seek to move body and spirit as an integrated unit.

9. There must be certainty in the movements. Will, as opposed to force, is applied to guide all body movements, making them continuous.

10. Seek serenity in activity. The perfect state to achieve is that of inner serenity and outer activity.

Sinking

This term refers to sending the essential energy, the qi (chi), to the dantian, where it can gather together more energy and become the force behind all of the movements. The dantian is divided into the lower abdomen, which controls sexuality; the middle abdomen, which is concerned with the heart and respiratory system; and the upper dantian, better known as the third eye, which governs energy and consciousness.

The benefits

Many people join tai chi classes to improve their health and spiritual state. However, tai chi also offers an element of self-protection, since the world is understood as a changing interplay of various forces. The theory is that people must realize their nature, and endure. The ideal for survival is integrity gained through persistence. The form of tai chi helps to train the body to be free, to learn a keen awareness of sensation and an intimate knowledge of a life force. In pursuit of power, the tai chi practitioner learns to yield rather than resist.

All forms of tai chi are designed to tap into the energy that runs throughout the body along pathways known as meridians. The points on these meridians are sometimes used by players as focal points through which energy can be directed, making a tai chi exponent extremely strong in will as well as body.

Results of research groups indicate that players of advanced ages who have been involved with tai chi all their lives show fewer signs of aging. It is ideal for older people because the movements are carried out in a slow and smooth manner.

The movements

In tai chi, the sequence of movements is learned and memorized. The form is specific in terms of direction and the shape of the body, and the placement of each part of the body. The sequences must be practiced daily until they become almost a natural habit.

The body is always upright in tai chi—unlike yoga, another Eastern relaxation technique. A practitioner of tai chi has to imagine his or her body's skeleton hanging from the crown of the head, completely relaxed through each of the joints. The weight of the body sinks downward through the legs and the feet, in a physical sense, placing roots in the ground. Stillness is at the center of tai chi and all movements start from this stillness.

Learning tai chi

The art of tai chi is not easy to learn. It may appear simple when an experienced player is seen going through the motions. However, it takes time and concentration to learn the sequences of movement and to become relaxed and completely coordinated while doing them. It is generally recognized that even if a student has learned all of the exterior movements and become a tai chi master, he or she will still continue to gain an internal spiritual knowledge.

Regular practice

A student of tai chi should first choose a suitable place to go through the sequences, and then ensure that practice can take place each day, preferably at the same time. Other, less important activities should not prevent regular practice.

The study is a long-term investment and the results gained are directly related to the amount of time and effort put into it. Initially the gains may be small, but gradually over the months and years, with regular practice, benefits will be noticed.

It is good to expand knowledge, and reading about the principles and philosophy of tai chi can be helpful. It is always a good idea to check the author's credentials, since there are many books on this subject and not all of them are authentic and useful. When someone practices tai chi it is natural to explore some of the other Eastern answers to Western stresses (see Shiatsu; Yoga).

Finding a teacher

One of the best ways to find a teacher is to contact a local martial arts school and ask for the name of a reputable teacher. Many community centers advertise the services of teachers.

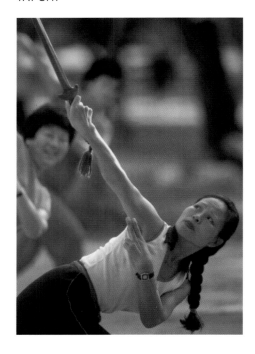

▲ *As in many other martial arts, swords are often part of the ceremonial art of tai chi. Here a woman with a wooden sword leads tai chi exercises in Victoria Park, Hong Kong.*

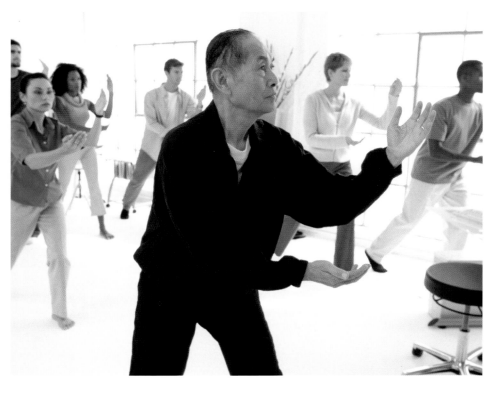

▲ *A tai chi session in the office at lunchtime can be a welcome and relaxing break from gazing at a computer screen.*

Before someone signs up for a class, he or she should ask to go along as an observer to get some experience of the teacher. It is important that a student of tai chi is satisfied with the way the teacher approaches the subject and feels comfortable with the relationship between them. If any unease is felt, it can be a barrier to learning. It is wise to ensure that the methods used conform to accepted tai chi principles.

Tai chi chuan

Chinese physical culture begins before history. A legendary philosopher of the 46th century B.C.E., who is believed to have created the original eight trigrams of the *I Ching*, ordered the performance of a Great Dance to help to cure his people of illness. This ancient combination of exercise with therapeutic and preventive medicine predates the beginning of the martial arts. As early as 190 C.E., a series of exercises based on the posture of animals was taught, and many of the steps of tai chi take their names from animals, both real and mythical. The expressions "carry the tiger to the mountain," "repulse the monkey," and "dance of the dragon" are a few of the names given to movements.

The person given credit for creating tai chi was a 14th-century Taoist monk by the name of Chang San-Feng, who recast the original elements of an exercise called Shao-Lin Ch'uan. He placed more of an emphasis on breathing and inner control. Apparently, tai chi was revealed to Chang during a midday meditation session. When he glanced out of a window he saw a magpie trying to attack a snake. The snake teased the bird, moving out of reach and curling around in spirals, which is a natural way for a snake to behave in the circumstances. From this spiraling snake, the inspiration for the essential spirit of tai chi was perceived and adopted. The earliest work is attributed to Chang. He states: "Ultimately, everything depends on one's will or mind and not on the external appearance of the movements." This leads us to assume that specific movements and the order of the sequence are not the most important factors. Another name associated with the origins of tai chi is that of Wang Chung-yueh, who lived in the 17th century. Wang is credited with having linked the 13 postures to create a continuous movement sequence. Two classic theoretical works are attributed to Wang Yang Lu-chu'an, an ambitious servant who became a well-known teacher in Peking. Tai chi is divided into different styles, identified by family names. The style called Yang, named after Yang Lu-chan, is now the most popular, and it is divided into two forms; long Yang and short Yang.

Benefits

Most practitioners of tai chi quickly find that they have a better sense of balance, greater flexibility of movement, improved circulation, and an improved sense of well-being; and many people find that they have lower blood pressure. Studies reveal that older people who have practiced tai chi enjoy better health than other people of the same age. With regard to breathing, cardiovascular functions, bone conditions, and general metabolism, they are in better condition than those who did not practice tai chi. The slow movements exercise the muscle fiber and the bones and improve the elasticity of the smooth vascular wall. This increases the circulation of the blood and stabilizes the vascular motor nerve.

See also: **Acupressure; Acupuncture; Alternative medicine; Feldenkrais method; Massage; Reflexology**

Taste

Questions and Answers

I recently fractured my skull. I have recovered but have almost completely lost my sense of taste. Have the nerves in my tongue been damaged?

Probably not. It is more likely that you sustained damage to the nasal twigs of the two olfactory nerves in the front of your brain. The loss of smell may not be obvious and in fact may be what you presume is a loss of taste. You can test this by seeing whether you can taste salt placed directly on your tongue. If it is your sense of smell that is missing the salt will be tasted normally.

I have noticed that since I quit smoking I can taste food much better. Does this mean that smoking affects the taste buds?

Smoking probably alters the ability of the taste buds to distinguish tastes to some extent, but most of your sense of taste probably has increased because your smell receptors have recovered from the smoke.

Do animals have a good sense of taste, and can they really tell the difference between the various foods offered to them?

Animals do have a good sense of taste, although it may not distinguish between different foods. However, some animals, deprived of certain vitamins or minerals, will seek out and eat foods that contain the missing substances.

Does a sense of taste improve with age?

Scientific tests show that it gets poorer as we get older, and by middle age is poor. However, experience allows older people to get more pleasure from a wider range of tastes and smells.

The word "taste" stands for discernment; yet in fact it is the most simple of the five senses, and we are capable of distinguishing only four basic taste sensations from our food and drink.

Of the five senses—sight, hearing, smell, taste, and touch—the sense of taste is the crudest. It is limited in both range and versatility and presents less information about the environment than any other sense. The exclusive role of the sense of taste is to select and appraise food and drink, a role that is helped by the more sensitive sense of smell, which adds information to the four basic tastes that the taste buds can recognize. Consequently, the loss of the sense of taste, for whatever reason, is less of a problem than the loss of the sense of smell (see Smell).

How food and drink are tasted

Like smell, the taste mechanism is triggered by the chemical content of substances in food and drink. Chemical particles are registered in the mouth and converted into nerve impulses that are then transmitted to the brain and interpreted. The taste buds are at the heart of this system. Studding the surface of the tongue (see Tongue) are many small projections called papillae. Inside the papillae are the taste buds. An adult has about 9,000 taste buds, mainly on the tongue's upper surface, but also on the palate, and even the throat (see Palate; Throat).

Each taste bud consists of groups of taste receptor cells, and each receptor cell has fine hairlike projections called microvilli, which are exposed on the surface of the tongue through fine pores in the surface of the papilla. The taste receptor cells link up with a network of nerve fibers. The design of this network is complex, since there is a great deal of linking between nerve fibers and receptor cells. Two different nerve bundles, which make up the facial nerve and the glossopharyngeal nerve, carry nerve impulses to the brain.

The taste buds respond to only four basic flavors: sweet, sour, salt, and bitter. The receptor sites for these tastes are located on different parts of the tongue. The buds that respond to sweet are at the tip of the tongue, whereas those specializing in salty, sour, and bitter flavors are located progressively farther back. Odor and some other stimuli combine with the four crude flavors to produce more subtle taste sensations.

How the taste buds respond to the chemicals in food and initiate nerve impulses to the brain is not fully understood, but in order to be tasted, the chemicals must be in liquid form. Dry food gives little immediate sensation of taste, and acquires its taste only after being dissolved in saliva (see Saliva).

It is believed that chemicals in food can alter the electrical charge on the surface of the taste receptor cells, which in turn cause a nerve impulse to be generated in the nerve fibers (see Nervous System).

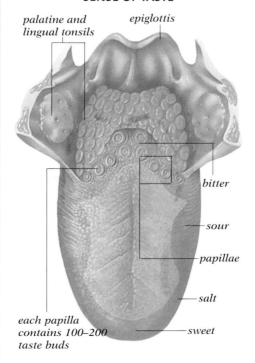

SENSE OF TASTE

palatine and lingual tonsils

epiglottis

bitter

sour

papillae

salt

sweet

each papilla contains 100–200 taste buds

◀ *The papillae on the tongue increase the area in contact with food and, except for those in the center, they contain numerous taste buds. The taste buds contain taste receptors that are distributed so that different parts of the tongue are sensitive to different tastes: sweet, salty, sour, or bitter.*

CROSS SECTION THROUGH THE TONGUE

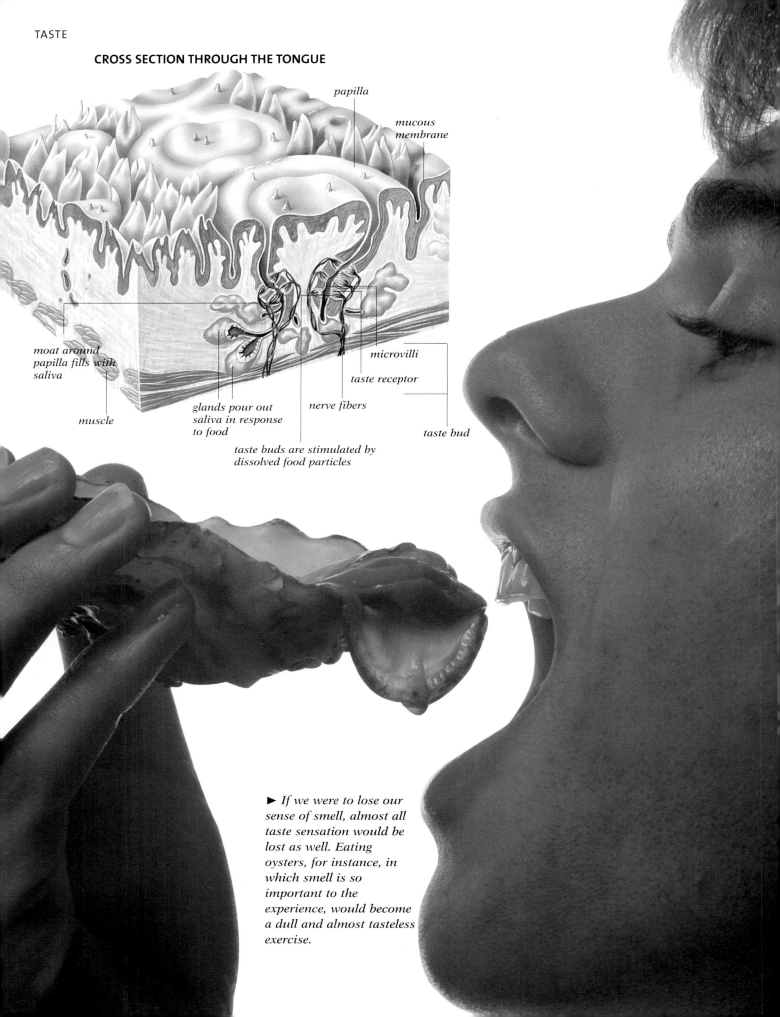

papilla

mucous membrane

moat around papilla fills with saliva

muscle

glands pour out saliva in response to food

nerve fibers

microvilli

taste receptor

taste bud

taste buds are stimulated by dissolved food particles

▶ *If we were to lose our sense of smell, almost all taste sensation would be lost as well. Eating oysters, for instance, in which smell is so important to the experience, would become a dull and almost tasteless exercise.*

Analysis of taste by the brain

The two nerves carrying taste impulses from the tongue (the facial nerve and the glossopharyngeal nerve) first pass an impulse to specialized cells in the brain stem. This area of the brain stem also acts as the first stop for other sensations coming from the mouth. After initial processing in the brain stem center, taste impulses are transferred through a second set of fibers to the other side of the brain stem and ascend to the thalamus. Here there is another relay, where further analysis of the taste impulses is carried out before information is passed to the part of the cerebral cortex participating in the actual conscious perception of taste.

The cortex also deals with other sensations, such as texture and temperature, which are transmitted from the tongue. These sensations are probably mixed with the basic taste sensations from the tongue, and so produce the subtle sensations with which we are familiar when we eat.

The analysis of the food eaten, carried out in the lower part of the parietal lobe in the cortex, is further influenced by smell information being analyzed in the nearby temporal lobe. Much of the refinements of taste sensation are due to smell sensations.

How sensitive are the taste buds?

Compared with other senses (in particular smell), taste is not very sensitive. It has been estimated that a person needs 25,000 times as much of a substance in the mouth to taste it as is needed by the smell receptors to smell it. However, despite this insensitivity, the combination of the four types of taste buds responding to the basic tastes of salty, sour, bitter, or sweet enables a wide range of sensations to be determined as the brain analyzes the relative strength of the basic flavors. Some of the stronger tastes, such as the hot flavor of spicy food, are experienced through stimulation of pain-sensitive nerve endings in the tongue.

What can go wrong?

Loss of taste usually comes about from a problem in the facial nerve. This nerve is connected to the muscles of the face, but a small branch carries the taste fibers from the front two-thirds of the tongue. For the part of the nerve involved in taste to become affected, the nerve must be damaged before the branch. This branch occurs just before the facial nerve passes near the eardrum. When frequent ear infections were common before the advent of antibiotics, operations had to be performed for mastoiditis and the facial nerve was frequently damaged (see Mastoiditis).

However, even when the nerve on one side of the face is severely affected, the other side will continue to send taste information to the brain. If the nerve that connects to the back third of the tongue is also damaged, there may be considerable loss of taste.

Taste may also be affected in a condition called Bell's palsy, in which the facial nerve becomes inactive quite suddenly owing to a variety of conditions, such as infections, tumors, herpes simplex, and meningitis. It is very rare for all taste nerves to be affected at the same time; complete taste loss is very rare.

It is much more common for people who have lost their sense of smell on both sides (for example, as the result of a head injury) to complain of loss or reduction in their sense of taste. This is because without the sense of smell, subtler refinements of taste are lost.

Unpleasant alterations in taste

It is common for people suffering from depression to complain of unpleasant tastes in the mouth. The cause of this is not clear, but it may be related to the close relationship of taste and smell. Smell-analyzing centers of the brain have close connections with the emotional circuitry of the limbic system, and it has been suggested that certain moods can conjure up tastes and smells. Another type of unpleasant taste occurs in some people as an aura or warning sensation before an epileptic fit. This usually means that the abnormal electrical activity causing the fit is centered either low in the parietal lobe or in the neighboring temporal lobe.

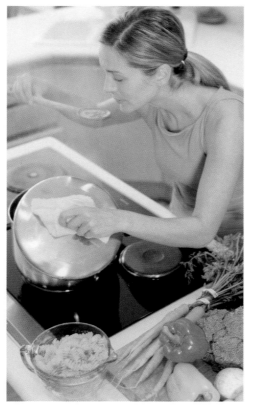

▲ As well as enjoying the delicious taste, part of the pleasure of eating sweet corn is experiencing the crunchy texture and smell of the cooked corn. Eating the corn alfresco is also part of the fun.

▲ One of the cook's tasks is to ensure that the food tastes good and is appropriately seasoned. Tasting a dish during its cooking time can test these criteria and also test for doneness.

See also: **Brain; Epilepsy**

Tattooing

Could I get blood poisoning from a tattoo?

Not if the tattooing has been done by a professional who took antiseptic precautions. However, there is a risk of hepatitis leading to jaundice if inadequate sterilizing methods are used. It is standard procedure in some hospitals to ask if you have had a recent tattoo so that your blood can be checked for the hepatitis virus before any surgery.

Why do tattoos fade with time?

The black pigment used in tattooing is relatively indelible, but the yellow, green, and red pigments are not permanent and gradually fade. Permanence also depends on the method used. The older, hand-pricked designs went deeper into the skin and lasted longer than those applied with an electrical instrument.

Can tattooing cause dermatitis?

Modern tattoo pigments are virtually nontoxic and should not cause a skin reaction. Older pigments, however, which are still occasionally used, may cause allergies. This is true of red and yellow pigments, which contain cadmium and cinnabar. An allergic reaction takes the form of a rash in the red and yellow area of the tattoo, and may spread to other parts of the body. To avoid a recurrence, the affected part of the tattoo would have to be removed.

I was tattooed as a teenager. Can I have the tattoo removed?

Yes, if it is not too large, but the procedure is costly and time-consuming. For small tattoos it is easier to have the area cut out. Larger tattoos may be removed by dermabrasion (high-speed sanding of the skin) or by laser treatment.

A spur-of-the-moment decision to have a tattoo can have a lifelong effect, and many people later regret the decision. The removal of a tattoo is never entirely satisfactory, and may be both painful and expensive.

The history of tattooing is a very ancient one. However, the origins of modern Western tattooing began in the British navy in the late 18th century, when sailors adopted the practice from South Sea islanders. In the 21st century, tattooing is still popular in the armed forces, and has been adopted by many young people as a fashion statement or a symbol of rebellion, and by street culture in general.

Owing to the increased sophistication of the instruments used and the strict regulation of tattooists, the health risks of tattooing are now minimal. The risks of blood poisoning (see Blood Poisoning) and of syphilis (see Syphilis), which used to be common complications, are now very small, provided that aseptic precautions are taken. However, there still seems to be a slight but significant risk of hepatitis (see Hepatitis) and AIDS following the procedure.

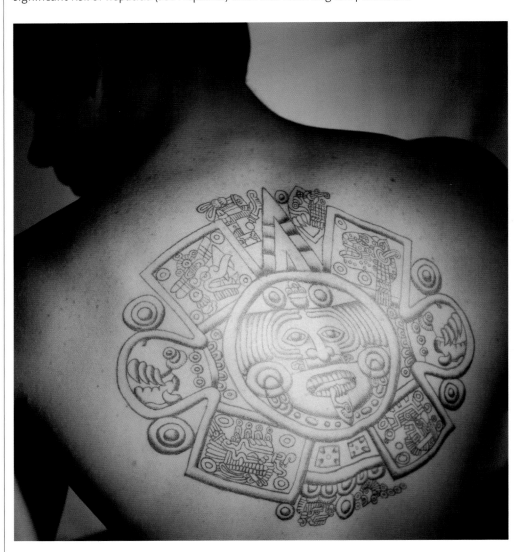

▲ *Tattoos can be simple images, or incredibly detailed, as shown in this example—a man with an Aztec calendar tattooed on his back.*

How tattooing is done

Techniques used to vary considerably but are now becoming much more standardized. Most tattooists first draw an outline of the design on the skin using transfers or stencils. The design is tattooed into the skin in black, and the colors are filled in afterward. The electrical tool used consists of a number of vibrating needles lying parallel inside a metal tube. Ink is inserted into the lower layer of skin (the dermis) by the pricking action of the needles. If ink was instead introduced into the surface layer of the skin, where cells are constantly being shed, it would soon disappear.

The discomfort of the procedure depends on the sensitivity of the area being tattooed. The skin over bony areas and the chest and abdomen is particularly sensitive. The sensation varies among individuals; to some people, being tattooed feels like a tickle, while to others it is a painful scratch. The initial outlining of an image is usually more painful than the filling in.

Aseptic precautions are necessary to prevent the complications of infection. The skin is cleansed with antiseptic and, if necessary, the area is shaved. The needles are sterilized after each client, and all the instruments are stored in sterile conditions.

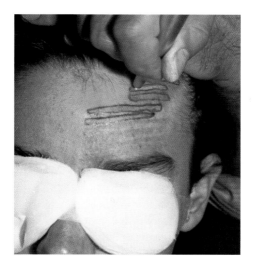

▲ *The most effective method of tattoo removal is laser treatment. The pigment is painlessly vaporized, and the slow process of healing is thereby avoided.*

After the tattoo is finished, it will be tender and sensitive. A dressing is applied for a couple of days, while a scab forms. This falls off to reveal the tattoo. The amount of bleeding should be minimal, but it does vary to a certain extent, possibly in relation to the bluntness of the needles used.

Removal of tattoos

The removal of tattoos is usually done by dermatologists or plastic surgeons. There are various methods of removal, but none is entirely satisfactory.

The most simple method, if the tattoo is small enough, is to cut out the tattooed area and to stitch the gap in the skin. Larger areas may also be cut out, but skin grafting may be necessary to close the wound (see Grafting). This method is time-consuming and may require time away from work.

Another type of treatment to remove a tattoo is dermabrasion, which is a technique of rubbing the skin with an abrasive instrument to create a deep graze. This is fairly painful and takes several months to complete. When the pigment in the skin has been removed, the body's cells start a process of inflammation and healing.

Laser treatment is the best method of tattoo removal, and has the advantage of being painless. The pigment in the skin absorbs the energy of the laser beam and is vaporized by it while the normal skin remains unaffected (see Lasers).

Finally, a tattooist may be willing to alter a design to make it more acceptable, although tattooists are traditionally reluctant to offer their services for the removal of tattoos.

Complications

Today the only serious risk of being tattooed is that of catching hepatitis and AIDS, and this is minimal when there is careful attention to aseptic techniques, though cases do occur. Infection due to ordinary bacteria is less of a problem, since most infections can be treated with antibiotics (see Antibiotics).

A less common problem is allergy to the colored pigments, particularly the red and yellow ones (see Allergies). Red pigments are often based on mercury, which can cause severe allergies even after many years. If this happens the tattoo may have to be removed. Modern pigments are less likely to cause this problem, but tattooists often prefer to use old, well-tried kinds.

Some skin diseases show a preference for tattooed skin, and may appear or worsen after tattooing (see Skin and Skin Diseases). Psoriasis and warts are examples of this (see Psoriasis; Warts).

Medical uses of tattoos

Tattoos may be used in the treatment of certain medical conditions. For example, after reconstructive surgery to the lips following an injury, normal lip color can be simulated by tattooing. Similarly, the pigmented area around the nipples can be imitated when breast reconstruction has been performed.

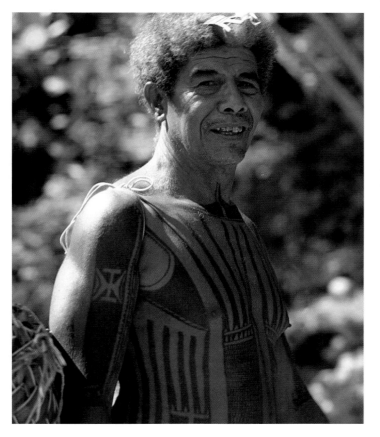

▲ *Many native peoples, the Polynesians among them, have long traditions of tattooing.*

See also: **Healing; Inflammation**

Tay-Sachs disease

This tragic condition is a genetic disorder affecting the nervous system of young children. It usually leads to death by age three. Members of families which might be affected should be aware of all the implications.

Questions and Answers

My husband and I are Jewish and there is a family history of Tay-Sachs disease. I want to know more about this condition. Can you explain what actually happens in the brains of affected children?

All nerve fibers have insulating fatty sheaths that are essential for their normal function. These fatty sheaths contain complex sugar-fat compounds called gangliosides. To form normal gangliosides an enzyme called hexosaminidase is necessary. In Tay-Sachs disease the gene for this enzyme is defective (mutated), so no hexosaminidase is produced. The result is a massive accumulation in the brain and peripheral nerves of an abnormal ganglioside called ganglioside GM2 . The rising quantity of this progressively destroys nerve tissue function.

Is the genetic defect inherited?

The defect is on chromosome number 15. Chromosomes, and therefore genes, come in pairs, one from the mother and one from the father. If the child has inherited a normal gene and a mutated gene there will be no problem. The normal gene will produce enough hexosaminidase to prevent the abnormal ganglioside from accumulating in the nervous system. If both genes have the mutation, none of the enzyme will be produced and the child will have the disease. This is called recessive inheritance.

How can a child have both genes affected if neither parent has the disease?

In this case, both parents would have to be carriers, each having one normal gene and one mutated gene. Unfortunately, among Ashkenazi Jews the mutation is quite common, so the chance that two mutated genes will come together is fairly high.

Tay-Sachs disease is a genetic disorder of nervous tissue, due to the absence of a vital enzyme. The lack of this enzyme leads to the accumulation of abnormal material called ganglioside GM2 in nerve fibers. The disease starts early in life and progressively destroys the function of nerve tissue wherever it occurs in the body. There is no treatment, so prevention is essential.

Symptoms

An affected baby appears normal at birth but by the age of three to six months there is obviously increasing muscle weakness. Even before this, an examination of the retinas with an ophthalmoscope may show a unique sign—the appearance of a bright cherry-red spot in the central area (the macula). As the motor weakness progresses to paralysis it becomes apparent that the child is showing no interest in the outside world. Soon seizures occur and there are clear indications of both deafness and blindness. Enlargement of the head occurs as a result of the buildup of ganglioside GM2 in the brain.

By about 18 months of age the baby is no longer responding to any external stimuli and the face has acquired a doll-like appearance. Seizures become more frequent and severe and the child lapses into a vegetative state with muscular rigidity and indications that the higher functions of the brain are no longer operating. All awareness has been lost and the child usually dies before he or she is three to five years old.

The diagnosis is initially based on the family history of the disease and the retinal appearance, but it may be confirmed by brain and blood cell analysis to detect the absence of the enzyme hexosaminidase.

Inheritance

Tay-Sachs disease is a recessive genetic disorder due to a mutation in a gene on chromosome 15. For the disease to occur the baby must inherit the mutated gene from both mother and father. The incidence of the disease among Ashkenazi Jews is around one in 2,000, and there is roughly a one in 30 chance that any such person, male or female, will carry the gene for the disease. Carriers of the mutated gene show no abnormality, but if two carriers marry, the chance with each pregnancy of having a child with Tay-Sachs disease is one in four (see Heredity).

A family history of disease is a clear indication that any direct descendant of either of the parents of a child with Tay-Sachs may be carrying the gene mutation. Whether or not such a person actually is a carrier can be determined by DNA testing.

Carriers who propose to marry should always receive expert genetic counseling and should be fully aware of the risks. If, in spite of such awareness, a pregnancy occurs, the fetus can be tested by chorionic villus sampling to check whether both genes are mutated. In this event, the parents can be offered the option of termination of the pregnancy while it is still in an embryonic stage.

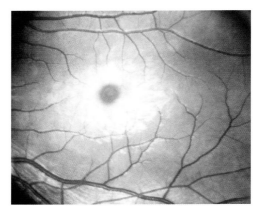

▲ *This picture shows the retinal deterioration that is typical of Tay Sachs disease. Sufferers eventually go blind.*

See also: **Genetic diseases and disorders; Genetic engineering; Genetics**

Teeth and teething

Everyone has two sets of teeth during his or her lifetime; the second set replaces the first throughout childhood. The function of teeth is to bite off pieces of food and grind them so they can be swallowed easily before digestion.

Why do some people have crooked teeth?

The development of the teeth and jaws is mainly controlled by inherited genetic factors. Each individual, however, has a unique assortment of genes and it is possible, for example, for a child to inherit large teeth from one parent and small jaws from the other, leading to overcrowding. However, teeth in irregular positions can often be aligned and made to bite together by using orthodontic appliances.

Does an impacted wisdom tooth always have to be removed?

An impacted wisdom tooth is unable to grow properly because its path is blocked, usually by the tooth in front. Some impacted wisdom teeth are highly prone to infection, especially those that are only partially through the gum. Such teeth are best removed. However, very deeply placed wisdom teeth may be best left alone if their removal requires the loss of an excessive amount of bone. Some impacted wisdom teeth, when developing, may overcrowd the incisors and should be removed. Your orthodontist will decide on the best treatment.

My niece was born with a tooth that had to be removed. Will she have a missing baby tooth when her teeth come through?

About one baby in 5,000 is born with one or two teeth already present in the mouth—Julius Caesar and Napoleon, for example, are both reputed to have had this distinction. It sometimes runs in families. These teeth are not fully formed and will fall out; occasionally, however, they present a danger of choking the baby, and so it is better to have them removed. The teeth will develop normally later on.

The teeth are hard, bonelike structures implanted in the sockets of the jaws. Two successive sets occur in a lifetime. Each tooth consists of two parts: the crown, which is visible in the mouth; and the root, which is embedded in the jawbone. The roots of the teeth are usually longer than the crowns. Front teeth have one root; those placed further back generally have two or three roots.

The major structural element of a tooth is composed of a calcified tissue known as dentine. Dentine is a hard, bonelike material that contains living cells. It is a sensitive tissue and gives the sensation of pain when stimulated either thermally or by chemical means. The dentine of the crown is covered by a protective layer of enamel, an extremely hard, cell-free, insensitive tissue. The root is covered with a layer of cementum, a substance similar to dentine, which helps anchor the tooth in its socket. The center of the tooth is a hollow chamber filled with a sensitive connective tissue known as dental pulp. This extends from within the crown right down to the end of the root, which is open at its deepest part. Through this opening, minute blood vessels and nerves run into the pulp chamber.

Each tooth is attached by its root to the jawbone; the part of the jaw that supports the teeth is known as the alveolar process. The mode of attachment is complex; teeth are attached to the jaw by the periodontal ligament. This consists of a series of tough collagen fibers that run from the cementum covering the root to the adjacent alveolar bone. These fibers are interspersed with connective tissue, which also contains blood vessels and nerve fibers. This method of attaching the teeth allows a very small degree of natural mobility. This serves as a buffer that may protect the teeth and bone from damage when biting. At the neck of the tooth where the crown and root merge, a cuff of gum bonded tight to the tooth protects underlying supporting tissues from infection and other harmful influences (see Gums and Gum Diseases).

Types of teeth

There are two series of human teeth. Deciduous teeth are those present during childhood and are all usually shed. Deciduous teeth can be divided into three categories: incisors, canines, and molars. The permanent teeth are those that replace and extend the initial series. They are the same types as the deciduous teeth, but in addition there is a further category known as the premolars, which are intermediate, in form and position, between canines and molars. Incisors have a narrow, bladelike incised edge. The incisors in opposite jaws work by shearing past each other like scissor blades. Canines

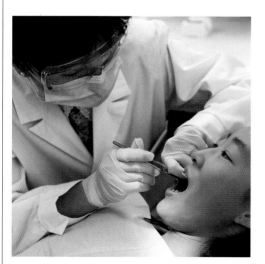
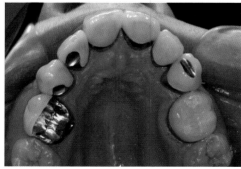

▲ *Dental decay can occur anywhere in a tooth and fillings will be the eventual result. To avoid this, it is important to take care of the teeth and visit a dentist regularly.*

Questions and Answers

I broke my front teeth in a car accident. Can they be repaired?

If only a small piece of enamel is broken off, then the sharp edges can be smoothed. If much of the tooth is missing, the tooth can be repaired by using a filling material bonded to the rest of the tooth, or a crown can be fitted. If the root of the tooth has been fractured, usually the tooth is extracted and replaced.

When milk teeth decay, why are they filled if they are going to fall out anyway?

It is usually preferable to fill them rather than extract them, since the early loss of milk teeth may cause the permanent teeth to drift into incorrect positions. Removal of teeth at the first signs of dental disease may make a child think that tooth loss is inevitable, and discourage the child from taking care of the teeth.

My son had a convulsion and then a high temperature. I thought it was due to teething, but my doctor sent him to the hospital. Was this necessary?

Teething does not cause high temperatures or any serious illnesses, although a child may be teething at the same time as he or she develops an illness. Your doctor was aware of this and wanted to ensure that there was no other cause for your son's fever and convulsion.

Should I give my baby fluoride tablets, which I've heard prevent tooth decay?

There is substantial evidence that the addition of fluoride to toothpaste and to water that contains a low level of natural fluoride helps prevent tooth decay, particularly in children. It may be a good idea to give your baby tablets if you live in an area where there is no extra fluoride in the water supply, but talk to your dentist and doctor before you go ahead with it.

DECIDUOUS (BABY) AND PERMANENT TEETH

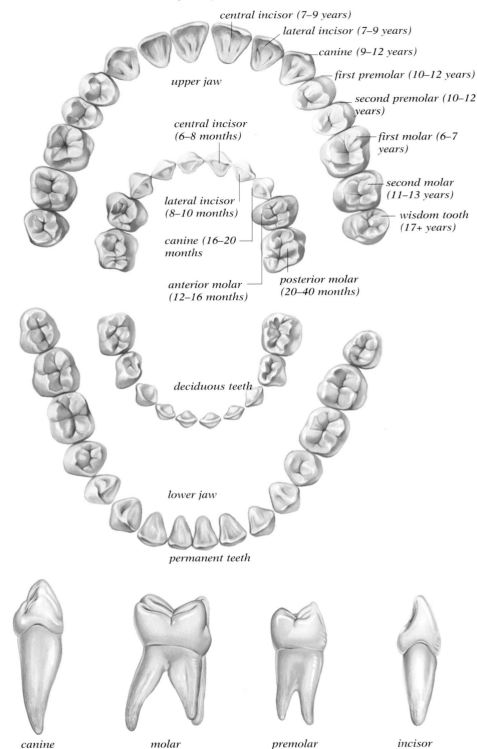

central incisor (7–9 years)
lateral incisor (7–9 years)
canine (9–12 years)
first premolar (10–12 years)
second premolar (10–12 years)
first molar (6–7 years)
second molar (11–13 years)
wisdom tooth (17+ years)

upper jaw

central incisor (6–8 months)
lateral incisor (8–10 months)
canine (16–20 months
anterior molar (12–16 months)
posterior molar (20–40 months)

deciduous teeth

lower jaw

permanent teeth

canine   molar   premolar   incisor

In theory we all have 32 permanent teeth. The arrangement of these is exactly the same in the upper and lower jaws. In each jaw there are 4 incisors, 2 canines, 4 premolars, and 6 molars—16 in total. Babies and young children have only 20 deciduous teeth. Again, in each jaw there are 4 incisors, 2 canines, and 4 molars—10 in all. Incisors cut food; canines tear it; and molars and premolars grind it. As human beings have evolved, teeth have changed; canines have become far less pointed, and many people never develop any wisdom teeth.

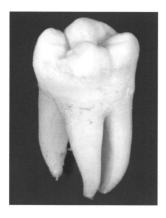 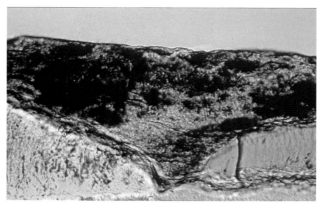

▲ *Each tooth consists of several layers: a stout shell of dentine (colored blue and yellow); cement covering the root (blue); and the crown's protective layer of enamel (yellow). The brown is plaque.*

ingrowths into the tissue that the epithelium covers. These buds then become bell-shaped and gradually grow to map out the shape of the eventual junction between the enamel and dentine. Some cells form the dentine; others give rise to the enamel itself.

The edges of the bell continue to grow deeper and eventually map out the entire roots of the teeth, although this process is not complete until after about one year. At birth the only sign of the occlusion is provided by gum pads, which are thickened bands of gum tissue. Around the age of six months, the first of the lower incisors pushes through the gum, a process known as dental eruption. The age at which this occurs is variable: a few babies have teeth at birth; in others they may not emerge until age one.

and pointed teeth are used for a tearing action; molars and premolars are effective at grinding food rather than cutting it.

Teeth form an even, oval-shaped arch, with the incisors at the front and the canines, premolars, and molars progressively placed farther back. The dental arches normally fit together in such a way that, on biting, the teeth opposite interlock with each other.

Development of teeth

The first sign of the development of the teeth occurs when the fetus is only six weeks old (see Fetus). At this stage the epithelial (lining) cells of the primitive mouth increase in number and form a thick band that has the shape of the dental arch. At a series of points corresponding to individual teeth, this band produces budlike

After the lower incisors have emerged, the upper incisors begin to erupt, and these are followed by the canines and molars, although the sequence may vary. Teething problems may be associated with any of the deciduous teeth. By age two and a half to three, the child will usually have a complete set of 20 milk teeth. Ideally, they should be spaced in a way that provides room for the larger permanent teeth. After age six, lower and then upper deciduous incisors become loose and are replaced by permanent teeth. The permanent molars develop behind the deciduous molars. The first permanent molars come through at age six, the second molars at age 12, and the third molars, or wisdom teeth, around age 18. There is, however, variation in the timing of the emergence of all the teeth. About 25 percent of people never develop one or more wisdom teeth. The reason may be

▼ *A dentist shows a woman an impression of her upper jaw; an impression is taken in preparation for making a crown.*

▼ *If teeth are crooked, spaced, or protruding, orthodontic appliances can be fitted.*

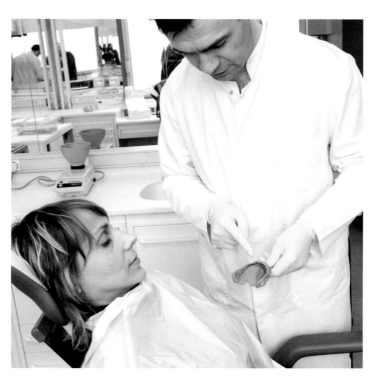 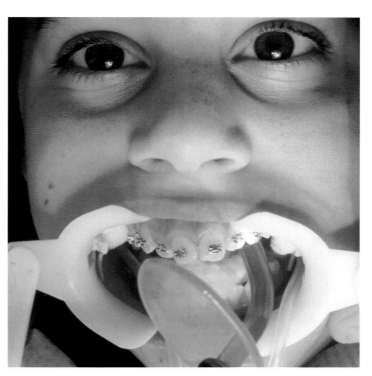

CROSS SECTION OF A MOLAR

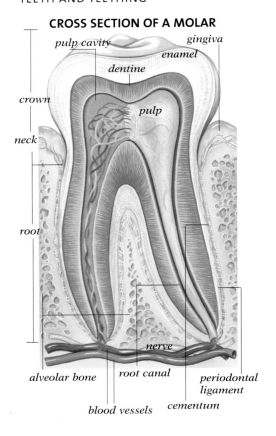

pulp cavity
gingiva
enamel
dentine
crown
pulp
neck
root
nerve
alveolar bone
root canal
periodontal ligament
blood vessels
cementum

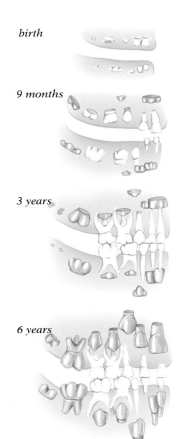

birth

9 months

3 years

6 years

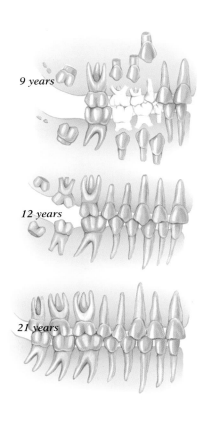

9 years

12 years

21 years

▲ A cross section of a molar shows the soft pulp where nerves and blood vessels are located. Dentin is the sensitive tissue around the pulp. Enamel covers the tooth above the gum; below the gum, cementum is the outer layer of the tooth.

▲ The deciduous teeth erupt at about six months; these are the central incisors. The first permanent teeth are molars, at age six. By the early twenties, everyone normally has a full set of teeth.

that the jaw is smaller, so the number of teeth has decreased. Some wisdom teeth never erupt through the gum and in 50 percent of people they become impacted and have to be removed.

Changes in teeth arrangement

The part of the jaw that supports the milk teeth increases very little in size from the age when all the milk teeth have erupted. It is only when the large permanent incisors have erupted that the final form of the dental arches become apparent. The upper permanent incisors often appear out of proportion to the child's face, but this naturally becomes less apparent as the face grows while the teeth remain the same size. Any tendency for the upper incisor teeth to protrude becomes obvious only when the milk teeth are replaced. Similarly, crowding often becomes clear only when the permanent teeth have erupted. During the six years that it takes for the milk teeth to be entirely replaced by permanent teeth, a gap may appear between the upper incisors. This gap usually closes when permanent canines push the incisors together, but the alignment or bite may need orthodontic treatment to bring the teeth into line.

Tooth eruption and teething

Many babies suffer discomfort as each tooth breaks through. Sometimes, a baby whose new tooth is hurting develops a red, inflamed patch on the cheek, and the gum may become red. There is excessive drooling, rubbing of the mouth, and crying; the cheeks

may appear pinker than usual. Symptoms such as fever or diarrhea are unlikely to be due to teething, and if they persist, medical advice should be sought. When teething causes the baby distress, a number of measures can be adopted, such as giving the infant a teething ring, a hard pacifier, or a piece of raw carrot to suck or bite on. Candy must never be given; this will damage developing teeth. In some cases anesthetic cream can be applied on the child's sore gum, but it wears off quickly because a baby salivates so much.

Some babies may have problems. Sometimes a bluish swelling, called an eruption cyst, appears over a molar tooth before it erupts. This disappears once the tooth emerges and does not require treatment. Anodontia, a total absence of teeth, is very rare, although the absence of individual teeth is a phenomenon that commonly occurs in about 5 percent of people. Tooth development can be delayed in a number of diseases affecting growth; for example, rickets (see Rickets). Children with Down syndrome may also have delayed teeth (see Down Syndrome), but this is rare. Some babies are as old as 18 months when the teeth erupt.

Tooth color varies from brown to deep cream. If a pregnant woman or a baby gets tetracycline antibiotics, the drug may cause a brown discoloration (see Antibiotics). Sometimes the incisors are twinned (joined together), but the second incisors usually develop normally.

See also: **Blood; Mouth; Nervous system; Orthodontics**

Telemedicine

Is telemedicine about buying drugs over the Internet?

No. Telemedicine covers every aspect of the provision of health care in which distant communication is involved. This includes medical teleconsultation, teleradiology, teleconferencing, distance medical learning, and even the performing of surgical operations by a surgeon situated at a remote distance from the patient. Telemedicine makes access to experts easier. It broadens the scope of consultation and can save medical costs as well as the time of expensive professionals.

My wife is a physician and she has been talking a lot about Internet2. What is this?

When American scientists involved in developing new technologies studied the potentialities of the Internet they soon realized that it was too heavily loaded with E-commerce, E-mail, and other matter to be suitable for their purposes. A new broadband network, dedicated to their objectives, was necessary. Internet2 is such a network. Since 1996, it has now grown to include more than 200 universities and technological organizations and it has links with other UK and European high-speed networks. You can find out more about Internet2 at www.internet2.edu.

What has Internet2 to do with medicine?

High-speed, broadband multimedia communication is essential if telemedicine is to realize its full potential. The network must be secure, confidential, and reliable. If a surgical operation is performed by an expert in a different country, it would be disastrous if the teleconference to discuss a difficult case were interrupted.

With the growth of the Internet, and the extraordinary facilities that it provides for communication, it was inevitable that it should come to play an important part in the process of providing medical care. This contribution has proved larger than even the most optimistic pioneers anticipated.

Telemedicine can be defined as including any medical activity involving long-range communication, whether verbal, auditory, visual, tactile, or all of these things, between doctors and patients or between doctors and their medical or paramedical colleagues. Telemedicine also includes the acquisition of medical information by patients and other laypersons without the direct involvement of qualified medical staff.

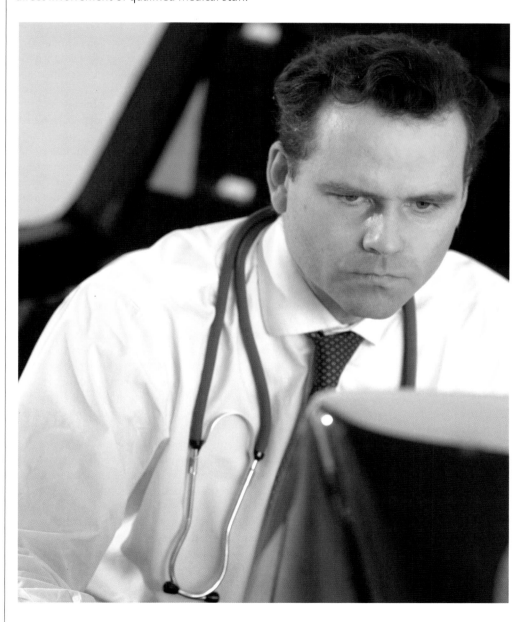

▲ *A doctor in a videoconference can discuss a medical case with a doctor in another country and show the other physician diagnostic images of the patient.*

Importantly, telemedicine is rapidly shifting the balance of power between health care professionals and the general public. So much specialist medical knowledge is now directly and easily available to nonmedical people that doctors are being challenged about whether they are, in fact, providing the best possible standard of care. This is a healthy development.

Medical information on the Internet

There is an enormous amount of medical information on the Internet, but it is not always easy to distinguish between authoritative, tested, reliable fact and uninformed foolishness. Unfortunately, because of the unrestricted access to Internet publication, some of what purports to be medical fact is nothing of the kind. Regrettably, the standards of medical ethics that govern the conduct of most qualified doctors do not necessarily apply to the authors of this material. As a result, much of it is motivated by commercial considerations rather than by the provisions of the Hippocratic oath. There are, however, many thousands of readily accessible and reliable professional medical web pages that can be used by anyone to obtain trustworthy medical updates.

Caution is needed in seeking medical information and advice from the Internet. It is easy to be misled by information published by impressive-sounding institutes and so-called colleges. Nothing should be regarded as authoritative unless it is produced by a recognized and formally licensed medical institution such as a known university, a teaching hospital, or a government-controlled research organization. Web publications from these sources are written by properly qualified authors of professional status, whose work is subjected to careful and critical review.

The safest approach is to limit browsing to the medical faculties of the better-known universities and government-sponsored health sites. The U.S. National Institutes of Health (www.nih.gov) and, in the UK, the National Health Service Direct (www.nhsdirect.nhs.uk) both publish large medical Websites for the nonmedical person. The full text of nearly all major general medical journals is accessible on the Internet, but because of the technical language these will often be difficult for laypeople to understand.

Teleconferencing

Teleconferencing has brought a whole new dimension into medical practice and has greatly increased its effectiveness. Doctors engaged in teleconferencing—usually to make decisions about difficult diagnoses or about the most effective form of treatment for particular cases—now have better resources than have ever been possible in the past. And the patient has the benefit of the combined knowledge and experience of a number of doctors with different areas of expertise. Instead of having to travel perhaps long distances, all these doctors can take part in a teleconference without leaving their offices.

During a teleconference doctors have immediate access to the patient's medical history and the results of all laboratory tests; they can see the patient, talk to him or her, and focus on any external physical signs; they can study digital X-ray or MRI images; they can watch a video of an endoscopic examination of the patient; they can see enlarged microscopic views of a biopsy taken from the patient; and they can then conduct a detailed discussion, referrring again to video material when necessary. A doctor can even look into a patient's ear remotely or listen to the heartbeat.

Telesurgery

An ever-increasing number of surgical operations are now being performed by endoscopic (keyhole) methods. Surgeons working in this way have a large and detailed monitor view of the operation field using miniaturized closed-circuit video systems and instruments controlled wholly from outside the patient's body. The instrumental controls can be electronically activated and need not be in the same room as the patient. They need not even be in the same country. To a surgeon performing such an operation at a remote distance the experience is the same as for one working close to the patient.

Endoscopic surgery calls for new skills and new designs of operating procedure, and many surgeons require training and experience in these new techniques. Telesurgical links are an ideal way of providing such training. Trainee surgeons have exactly the same view of the operation site and the instrument tips as the operator. They can even participate progressively in the operation.

An important element in telesurgery is tactile feedback—a technology known as haptics—by which the operator can feel the changing resistance to the manipulation of the instruments as he or she performs different procedures.

Teleradiology

Many hospitals have now completely abandoned the once standard practice of producing X-ray films by photographic methods and storing multiple serial films in thousands of large and heavy envelopes. Retrieval was slow, troublesome and expensive; films, or reports on them, were commonly lost; and problems of storage space had become acute. When the old system has been replaced by a purely digital system, in which high-resolution images are stored electronically on computer hard drives, all these problems are overcome. But there is another equally important consequence. Radiological images, whether X rays or CT, MRI, ultrasound, or PET scans, can be made immediately accessible to anyone anywhere in the world, and they can be made available, simultaneously, to any number of experts. Backup copies of the video files can be stored remotely in a small space.

Other areas of telemedicine

Telemedicine technology is used in prisons, when authorities do not wish to transport dangerous inmates to health facilities, and in hospices, enabling the nursing staff to consult with physicians without physically leaving the premises. More recently, some school health services are using the technology to allow nurses at schools to consult with physicians and get medical advice for students.

There is also an application for telemedicine technology for remote areas that do not have easy access to health care, and for underdeveloped countries. Home health care is another expanding area in this field, allowing homebound patients to have easy communication with doctors, therapists, and nurses.

Robotics equipment is being developed for telesurgery. This has particular application for the armed forces, because in a battlefield situation, a surgeon in one location can remotely control a robotic arm and instrument in another place. The technology is tested and used by some academic medical centers and also by some research bodies.

See also: **Health care system; Hospitals; Surgery**

Temperature

Does a high temperature help fight infection?

Yes. Bacteria that cause infections in humans have evolved to reproduce effectively at room temperature. They do so less well at other temperatures, so it is not always good to lower temperature. Unduly high temperature is dangerous and must be avoided.

My temperature always seems low. Is this a problem?

It is quite normal for your temperature to be a little lower than average. In fact, the normal range of temperature is quite wide, between 96° and 99°F (35.6° and 37.3°C).

During moderately hard exercise, does the body temperature rise?

Yes, but there is a wide difference between the temperatures of various parts of the body. Doctors refer to the core temperature; this is the presumed temperature inside the body, and is usually measured by taking the rectal temperature. The core temperature of someone doing hard exercise may be higher than normal; it can be as high as 102°F (39°C).

Is it common to take a rectal temperature?

It is often used for babies and small children and in adults in cases of hypothermia, since it is an accurate method. In such cases a low-reading thermometer is used. Rectal temperatures are taken in intensive care units, when an electronic probe gives a constant record of the temperature, which can be compared with a similar probe taped to the big toe. The difference between the two is an indication of how efficiently the heart is pumping blood.

The body's sophisticated temperature control mechanism is one of the major features that set humans aside from lower forms of life. The way that heat is produced and lost depends on a series of complex bodily functions.

Those who live in temperate climates often take very little notice of the temperature of their surroundings, yet the temperature of the environment is one of the most important factors in determining how people live.

The temperature of the outside world is very important in the way it affects our so-called internal environment. In a very advanced animal like a human, there are several sophisticated mechanisms that are designed to keep the internal environment balanced, despite any change

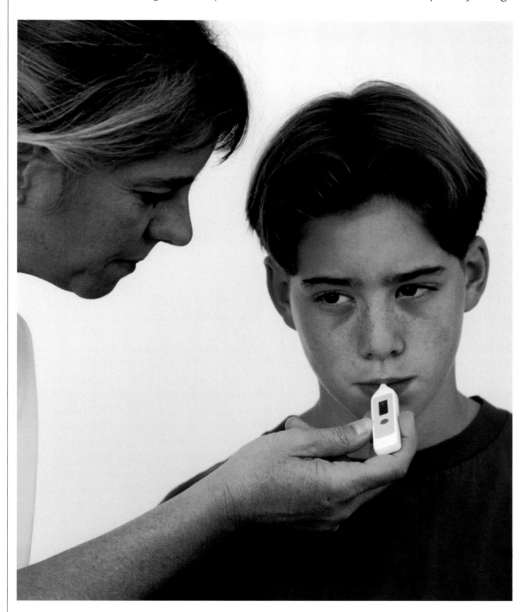

▲ *Temperature is measured by placing a thermometer in the mouth. In this case, a digital thermometer is used with a display that is easy to read.*

in the external conditions. The maintenance of a constant temperature, constant levels of salt and water in the tissues (see Salt), constant supplies of oxygen (see Oxygen), and a constant balance of the amount of acid and alkali in the body is controlled by a process called homeostasis. Temperature control is perhaps the most important element of the homeostatic mechanism.

If, for instance, the mechanism that regulates temperature were to break down or to start to work inefficiently, then a number of potentially fatal disorders could result (see Hypothermia).

Temperature control

All forms of life depend on chemical reactions and the enzymes that regulate their reaction rate (see Enzymes). It is the temperature at which these reactions take place that determines their speed and whether or not they happen quickly enough to be of use to the body. An internal temperature that is fixed within narrow limits ensures that chemical systems in the body work efficiently.

It is only the higher forms of life such as warm-blooded mammals or birds that can keep their internal temperatures constant within a very small range. This allows them an existence that is much less controlled by external circumstances than the lives of cold-blooded reptiles, whose less efficient chemical systems have to work over a much wider range of temperature.

How temperature control works

To enable the body to maintain a constant internal temperature during heat loss, the balance will be regained by the production

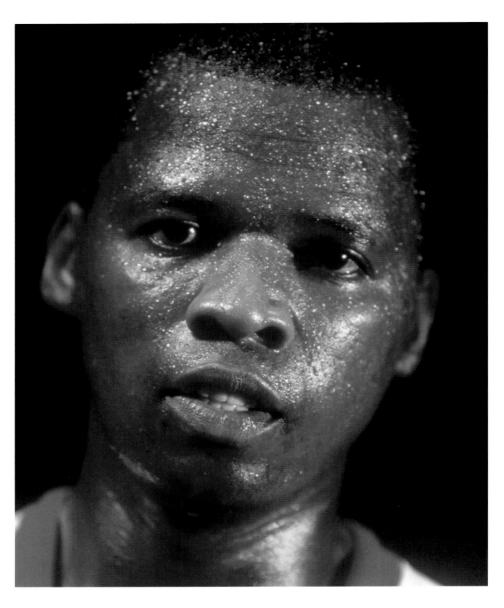

▲ *This basketball player is sweating profusely to stay cool after a strenuous game.*

of an equivalent amount of heat. If, on the other hand, a person is basking in hot sunshine, then heat is being absorbed by the body rather than being lost from it. In these circumstances, the body has to have an efficient way of losing heat.

The system of temperature control is one that determines that heat lost from the body must be made up, and heat gained must be reduced in order to maintain a stable temperature. The overall control of this temperature system is managed by the hypothalamus, the area at the base of the brain that governs so many of the body's vital functions (see Hypothalamus).

Heat production

When the body temperature starts to fall, there are a number of processes that the body can set in motion to produce more heat. However, certain mechanisms in the body already constantly produce heat, since every one of the body's many chemical reactions liberates some heat as it takes place. This is called the heat of metabolism, and the general rate at which these reactions take

place is called the metabolic rate. Although it cannot be controlled entirely by one organ, the metabolic rate is very closely related to the activity of the thyroid gland. An overactive thyroid will lead to a high metabolic rate, whereas an underactive thyroid causes a low metabolic rate. This close relationship between thyroid function and heat production explains why people who have an overactive thyroid are very intolerant of hot weather, and those who have an underactive thyroid feel the cold and so may be more prone to suffer from hypothermia (see Thyroid).

If the heat of metabolism is insufficient to meet the demands of the homeostatic control system, then the hypothalamus will increase the activity of the muscles by working particularly on the main postural muscles up and down the spine.

What happens first is an increase in the tone of the postural spinal muscles, so more energy is used by each muscle fiber, and more heat is generated. We are not aware that the hypothalamus is making these subtle alterations in the tone of the main postural muscles, but they are the most important way of making extra heat.

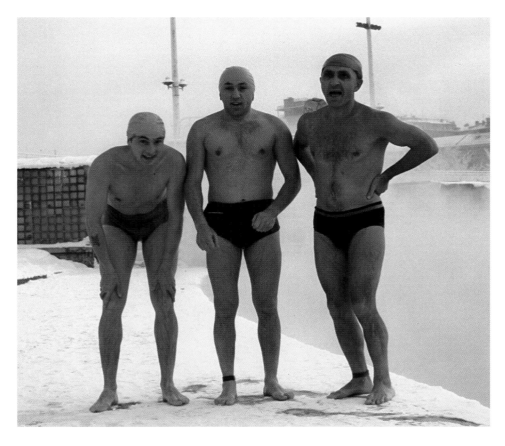

▲ *Even Russia's frozen winters can't deter these swimmers from taking the plunge.*

same person is standing in the hot sun, then the opposite will happen; heat will be radiating into him or her.

If the amount of blood, and therefore the amount of heat, that flows through the skin is increased, then the amount of heat lost by both convection and radiation will also increase. This increase in the flow of blood through the skin is in fact the main way in which the hypothalamus controls heat loss from the body.

Following an increase in the flow of blood to the skin in order to lose heat, there will of course be an increase in the amount of sweating (see Perspiration). The sweat glands work by liberating sweat onto the surface of the skin; the sweat is then evaporated with a consumption of heat in the same way that the evaporation of water from the lungs loses heat.

Most sweating takes place at a low level so that moisture is rarely noticed on the skin. However, when the system becomes overworked, and is therefore not working efficiently, sweat is clearly visible on the surface of the skin.

The efficiency of the function of sweating also depends on the humidity of the air. Humidity is the amount of water already present in the air in the form of water vapor. If someone sweats profusely when there is a lot of humidity, the sweat will not easily evaporate. This causes the body to be less efficient at losing heat than it should be (see Humidifiers).

If the hypothalamic alterations in the amount of tone in the postural muscles fail to produce enough heat, another familiar and obvious mechanism comes into play: shivering. Shivering works by setting up alternate contraction and relaxation in many muscles in the body. This action uses up energy and so starts to heat the body.

Heat loss

Just as the main way of gaining heat is not really obvious to us, so the main mechanisms by which heat is lost function without our being aware of them.

The body has a certain amount of heat that it cannot avoid losing. Food and drink may have to be warmed by the body to its own temperature, and in cold conditions we have to warm the air we breathe. As we breathe there is also some unavoidable loss of water, in the form of vapor, from the lungs (see Breathing). Such vaporization or evaporation of water uses up heat the same way as heat is used up in steam from boiling water.

Apart from the heat that is lost in these various ways in the gut and the lungs, another type of heat loss happens through the skin. There are two main ways of heat loss through the skin: convection and radiation. Convection is the system in which a fluid or gas moves from colder to warmer areas, carrying heat with it. In the case of the skin, it is usually cool air that moves across the surface of the skin and, as it does so, takes heat from the surface and carries it away from the body; the air becomes warmer in the process.

Radiation, on the other hand, is the way in which an electric fire produces heat, by pushing it out directly into the environment. In a cold climate a person will radiate quite a lot of heat; but when the

Measuring temperature

The main reason people want to measure body temperature is to see if we have a fever (see Fevers). The standard way of measuring temperature is with a thermometer.

In all older children and adults the way of taking a temperature is to place the thermometer under the tongue for about 90 seconds, and then to remove it and read it. In very small children or babies, there is a possibility of the thermometer's being bitten off in the mouth, so the temperature may be taken using an aural thermometer, which is placed gently into the child's ear. Other methods are taking the temperature under the armpit or in the rectum. To take an axillary (armpit) temperature, the thermometer is put into the armpit and kept there, with the arm pressed against the side, for about two minutes. The temperature will read slightly lower than an oral temperature. In a baby, a rectal temperature is best taken with the baby face downward on your knee. The thermometer should be held gently between the fingers, with its tip in the rectum and the hand flat on the buttocks. The reading will be slightly higher than an oral reading.

Medical thermometers have an interior kink in them so that the column of mercury, which shows the temperature, will not immediately fall back to room temperature when taken from the mouth. Once the temperature has been taken, a thermometer should always be shaken so that the column falls back down. The

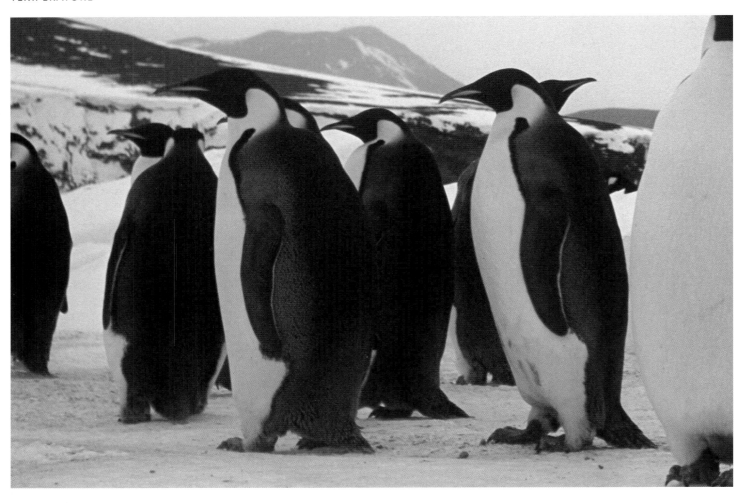

▲ *Warm-blooded animals like these emperor penguins are so well insulated by fat and feathers that they can live happily in the freezing conditions of Antarctica.*

▼ *Cold-blooded reptiles like crocodiles have to live in a climate that remains sufficiently hot so that their essential chemical functions are not switched off by the cold.*

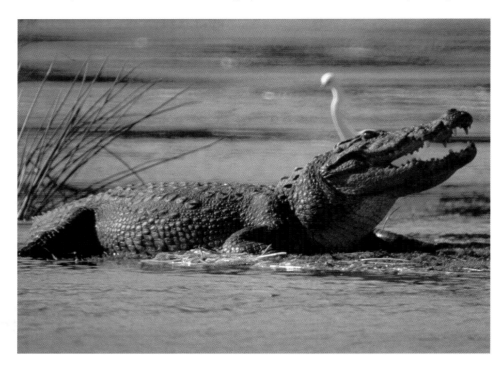

thermometer should be rinsed in cold water or alcohol, since hot water causes the mercury to expand and may break the thermometer.

As well as checking for possible fever, there are other reasons for taking a temperature, such as wishing to know if and when ovulation has occurred.

In intensive care units, a special instrument called a thermistor is used for measuring temperature. The thermistor checks if the heart is working hard enough, or whether it is failing to pump enough blood around the body. The temperature of the central part of the body is measured simultaneously with that of the big toe. A minor difference in temperature indicates a relative lack of blood being supplied to the peripheral areas.

See also: **Heat and heat disorders; Homeostasis; Metabolism; Muscles**

Tendons

Questions and Answers

Is it possible for tendons to be dislocated?

This is an unusual occurrence, but it can happen. Normally it is brought about by a sudden wrenching movement powerful enough to jolt a tendon out of the groove over a bone in which it runs. Treatment consists of manipulating the tendon back into its proper position.

My boyfriend accidentally cut through one of the tendons in his wrist. Will he be able to use his hand after the tendon has healed ?

In most cases it is possible to sew the cut ends of the tendon together again. This is usually successful in restoring full movement to the affected muscle on recovery. But the tendon may not be as strong as it was and its use may give rise to discomfort.

Do severed tendons ever heal naturally?

If the tendon is nicked or only partially severed, scar tissue will probably form to fill in the gap. If the tendon is completely severed, the two ends are likely either to spring apart because they are under tension, or separate when the muscle moves. Unless they are identified and deliberately sewn firmly together, healing is unlikely.

What is likely to cause actual damage to the tendons?

Sudden sharp strains or twisting pressures on a tendon are likely to tear some of the tendon fibers away from the bone to which they were anchored. Alternatively, repetition of a movement over a long period of time may use up all the lubricating fluid in the tendon sheath and thus give rise to the friction and inflammation of tenosynovitis.

Although very simple and apparently minor parts of the body's structure, tendons play a very important role in transmitting muscular power and enabling movement.

Tendons, or sinews, are vital to facilitating a wide variety of movements. A tendon is a very strong and tough band of fibrous connective tissue that joins the active section or body of a muscle to another part, usually a bone, which it is intended to move. The force of the contracting muscle fibers is concentrated in and transmitted through the tendon, achieving traction on the part concerned and thus making it move (see Body Structure; Bones; Muscles).

Tendons and muscles

Tendons are specialized extensions or prolongations of muscles. They are formed by the connective tissue, which binds the bundles of muscle fibers together, joining and extending beyond the muscles as a very tough, inelastic cord. They have very few nerve endings and, being essentially inactive tissues, little in the way of a blood supply. At one end they are formed from the belly of the muscle, and at the other they are very firmly tethered to the target bone, some of their fibers being actually embedded in the bone structure.

Location

Several tendons are located just beneath the surface of the skin, and so can be felt easily. For instance, the hamstring tendons, which control knee bending, are at the back of the knee.

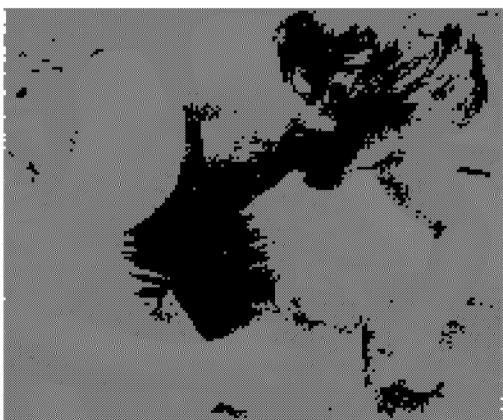

▲ *Should this man miss with his mallet, he could damage a tendon. In addition, regular use of certain muscles can cause tenosynovitis.*

TENDONS AND TENDON SHEATHS

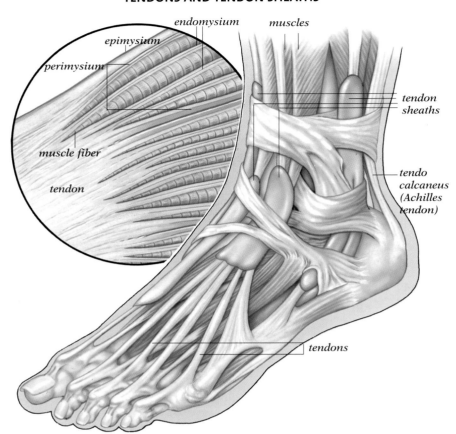

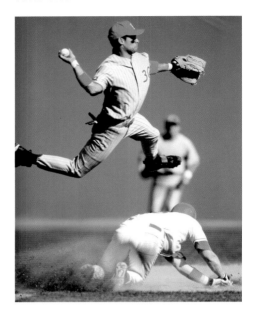

▲ *Tendons take fierce punishment during physical exertion.*

Because they take up much less space than muscles, tendons are also often found where there are a large number of joints to be moved in a relatively small space. Therefore both the backs and the fronts of the feet and the hands contain a whole array of different tendons (see Feet; Hand). The muscles that make these tendons work are sited in the arms and legs.

An unusual tendon is found in connection with the muscle tissue that forms the wall of the heart and brings about its pumping action. Thickened, fibrous connective tissue forms tough strips within the heart muscle, which give it a firmer structure as well as forming firm supporting rings at the points where the large blood vessels join the heart.

▲ *The membranes surrounding the muscles and muscle fibers (the endomysium, the perimysium, and the epimysium) join at the end of a muscle to form the tendon (inset above). Sheaths stop tendons from rubbing against other structures (above).*

Tenosynovitis

In order that they can move smoothly and without friction or the danger of abrasion, tendons are enclosed in sheaths at the point where they cross or are in close contact with other structures.

The tendon sheath is a double-walled sleeve designed to isolate, protect, and lubricate the tendon so that the possibility of damage from pressure or friction is reduced to a minimum. The space between the two layers of the tendon sheath contains fluid so that when the muscle is in action the two layers slide over each other like the parts of a well-oiled machine.

The human body, however, cannot sustain repeated movements in the same part of the body without sustaining damage in the form of inflammation, so rest periods are necessary for the lubricating fluid to be replenished. If this does not happen, and the system is run without adequate lubrication, the two layers of the tendon sheath begin to rub against each other and chafe. Continued movement will then be painful and cause a creaking sound called crepitus. This is the basis of the condition called tenosynovitis—inflammation of the tendon sheath. Any tendon sheath can be afflicted by this annoying and painful condition, which is common in keyboard operators, athletes, dancers, and others who use one particular set of muscles repeatedly. Sudden, unaccustomed use of a particular set of muscles is especially likely to cause tenosynovitis.

Injury

Virtually all the disorders of tendons are due to injury of one sort or another. A deep cut near the foot, ankle, hand, or wrist may sever one of the tendons that lie quite close to the surface.

It is usually possible to sew the two severed ends together, but there always remains the possibility of pain or some weakness of the muscle when it is used for a long time.

Extreme tension, overstretching, or sudden jerking on a tendon may damage it in a variety of ways. Some of the fibers of the tendon anchoring it to the bone become torn away from their moorings. The tendon itself is not really stretched, and only very rarely ruptured or snapped, since the force required to do this would already have pulled it away from the bone.

Injuries to tendons are usually treated with ice packs and rest, with the support of an elasticized bandage. Rather than exercise regularly, a gradual return to normal use is the best way to regain full use of the limb involved in the injury.

See also: **Exercise; Sports injury**

Tennis elbow

Questions and Answers

If I had tennis elbow, how would I recognize it?

You would have a dull ache around the elbow area and upper side of the forearm, with a particular tender spot on or near the bump that can be felt on the upper side of the elbow when the forearm is placed across the chest. Typing, using a squash or tennis racquet, or even picking up heavy objects may be painful.

How soon can one resume playing tennis after tennis elbow?

That depends on how serious the injury was; you should seek your doctor's advice. The symptoms vary from person to person. In mild cases, you may have to wait only a few days until the pain and stiffness subside, and resume the sport gradually. More serious cases may take longer. If you find that the tenderness returns whenever you play, consult your doctor as soon as possible.

I am due to play in a tennis tournament, but now have tennis elbow. What can I do?

Ask your doctor for a painkilling injection, but he or she may not be willing to give it. The danger is that you could seriously aggravate the injury and delay full healing for weeks or even months. As an alternative wear an elasticized bandage around the affected forearm to provide relief and reduce the chance of aggravating the injury. Ideally you should rest the arm for a few days.

Do you get tennis elbow only from playing tennis?

No. The injury is common in many sports, especially racquet sports, and also occurs as a result of doing other repetitive tasks, such as those involved in carpentry.

This painful muscle condition deserves its graphic name. Although athletes suffer from it, it can also be brought on by mundane activities such as wringing out wet clothing.

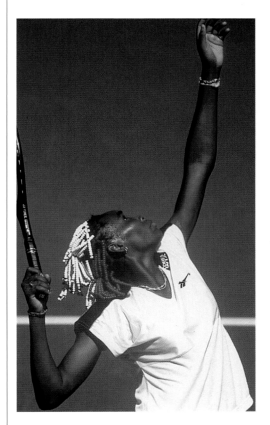

▲ *The flamboyant tennis star Venus Williams demonstrates her fluid service action, which requires healthy muscles.*

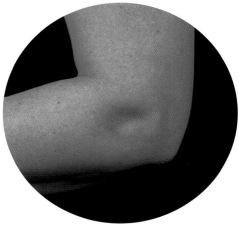

▲ *A case of tennis elbow.*

Tennis elbow is a common arm injury. Although it often develops during a game of tennis, it can also occur in other sports, and even as a result of nonsporting activities. The injury is not in fact to the elbow itself, but an inflammation of the tendon that attaches the muscles of the forearm to the bones of the upper arm (see Tendons). The muscles control movements of the wrist and fingers; that is why it is such a common injury among racket players. The elbow joint forms a pivot between the bone in the upper arm (humerus) and the two bones in the forearm. At the lower end of the humerus are two projections (epicondyles) to which forearm muscles are attached. The pain is due to small tears where the muscles join the lateral epicondyle.

The cause of the injury is vigorous or prolonged use of the forearm muscles, especially during sports such as tennis, squash, racquetball, and athletic throwing events. It can also be caused by wringing out wet clothing or using a carpentry tool such as a screwdriver.

Symptoms and treatment

Tennis elbow comes on gradually, and is made worse by activities that involve gripping something or picking up a heavy object such as a full kettle. A very tender spot can usually be felt at the site of the injury where the forearm muscles are attached to the lateral epicondyle, but pain and stiffness may sometimes extend over the whole of the upper side of the forearm.

Rest and a pain-relieving drug usually permit use of the affected arm within a few days. More persistent tennis elbow may be treated with a corticosteroid injection containing an anesthetic to reduce pain and tenderness during healing.

When the injury is severe and persistent, heat treatment and physical therapy are used. Some have found acupuncture helpful.

> **See also: Acupuncture; Bones; Muscles**

Tension

Is tension always a destructive force in humans?

Not at all. It is generally a constructive force stimulating resourcefulness and inventiveness, and biologically designed to promote survival. We would soon lose motivation without tension in our lives; and we would probably not survive for very long without it to stimulate us.

Is there any specific type of tension that is particularly insidious today?

One of the most insidious and serious features of life today is that it has become extremely difficult to achieve ordinary things like traveling to work, getting the groceries, driving the car, taking a bus or train, and many other common daily activities without becoming unwillingly involved in a web of hassles every day of our lives. These nonproductive conflicts give rise to high levels of tension for which there is no constructive outlet, and which are very potent forms of stress.

What defenses do people have against the buildup of tension?

Several. First, the example and encouragement of having handled problems successfully in the past, allied to the skills of one's particular trade. Second, the confidence that one is able to succeed, and an interest in doing so. Third, the defenses of escape, avoidance, and adaptability in leisure pursuits. Serious attempts at relaxation and a determination to avoid reacting to stressful events can be a great help. All of these must be utilized to the full whenever the going gets rough. Finally, there is the support of somebody close to us, not only in lending a sympathetic ear but also in helping us to keep things in perspective and in giving advice.

As an insidious component of modern life, tension can occur during even the most mundane everyday activities. Prolonged tension is a form of stress that in some people can trigger physical and psychiatric illness.

Tension and strain, in the emotional or mental rather than in the mechanical or physical sense, are major elements in the range of stressful influences that operate in modern life. Tension and strain are things that happen to all people, usually every day. They are the load, the pressure, the effect that is imposed on people by the inevitable confrontations that sometimes occur between them and their environment in terms of the other people, the things, and the circumstances that

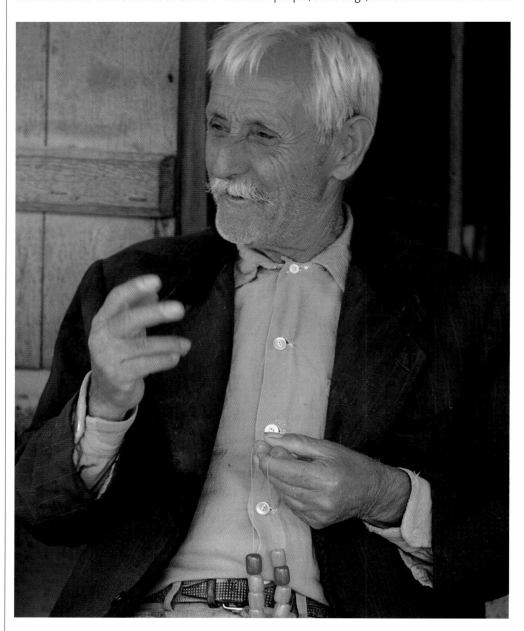

▲ *Worry beads are very popular with many different cultures. There is a traditional thought that "having something to do with your hands" can reduce tension.*

surround them. However, in some people the tension or strain becomes more than they can cope with and some sort of breakdown in health results (see Nervous Breakdown).

Causes of tension

Tension occurs for a variety of reasons and in a variety of ways. The most basic and intense tension results from situations where the expression of our instincts is inhibited. The universal, primary instincts are concerned with self-protection and preservation of life, obtaining food and drink, and reproduction (see Sex). These are regarded as the primary instincts, since without them and the driving force that they supply, both people as individuals and humankind as a species would perish. These are the things that, in most people, are inborn as driving forces that override all else.

The secondary instincts are not quite so demanding as the primary, and are not so vital to human survival.However, for most people they are vital to happiness. The first of them is the power instinct, which drives people to be competitive and ambitious, and to try to gain positions of superiority over others in terms of achievement, wealth, position, or title. The second is the herd instinct, which leads people to think and act in groups and communities. Finally, although this is denied by some psychologists, there is the spiritual instinct that urges people toward goals that are nonselfish, idealistic, and, at least materially, unrewarding. These primary and secondary instincts constitute the major basic driving forces in most people's lives; satisfying them without conflict or restraint gives people a sense of security and emotional happiness and contentment.

If, on the other hand, the achievement of their demands is made impossible or difficult, mental tension and pain result. This tension, if it is severe enough, will lead to some form of mental or physical stress illness. The likelihood of this depends on the extent to which the instinct concerned has been frustrated, the mental strength and capacity for adapting to a heavy tension load of the person involved, and whether or not an alternative area of satisfaction is available.

Many feelings that appear as tension are related to particular instincts. Fear, for example, is associated with concerns about self-preservation and security; anger with the need for confrontation and combat; loneliness with the desire for company and protection of the herd; appetite and hunger with the need for regular nourishment; sexual desire with the need to produce future generations. Therefore the satisfaction of instincts is associated with and results in pleasurable, happy feelings, while their frustration generally results in tension and unpleasant, painful feelings.

Conflict

However, the frustration of instincts and other desires leads not only to feelings of tension and unhappiness, but also to something that frequently accompanies tension—conflict. Tension and conflict, though born of frustration and dissatisfaction, are nevertheless the fundamental mainsprings of human endeavor and progress. They occur whenever what a person wants to do is not immediately possible, and they can result from a wide variety of circumstances. What a person wants to do may involve him or her in a collision course with another person after the same goal. Or it may be incompatible with the interests of the herd or the rules of the community in which he or she lives. Or it may represent a struggle with some limitation imposed by the body, such as illness or disability, or with an obstacle in the world surrounding him or her,

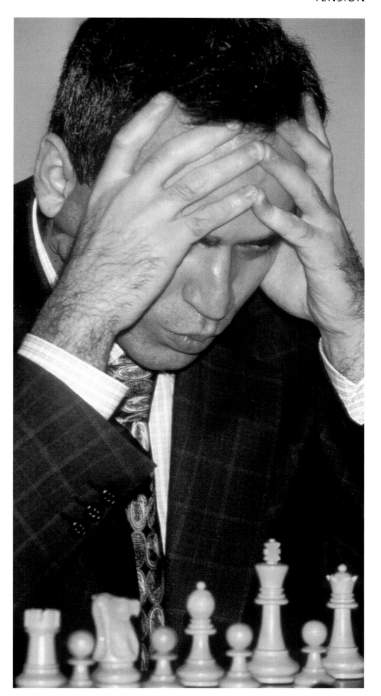

▲ *The tension inherent in playing a skilled game for very high stakes shows up only too clearly on the face of the brilliant chess player Garry Kasparov.*

such as drought or flood. Or the tension may be the result of the demands of rival instincts and emotions that are competing with each other for domination in the person.

There are four possible outcomes to a situation of tension conflict: the person may be successful and victorious; the person may decide to submit; the person may try to escape; or the tension may continue and interfere with the stability of the person's life, in the form of stress, indefinitely. Submission normally occurs when a person realizes that to continue the conflict is no longer in his or her

Questions and Answers

Do all people respond to tension in the same way?

No, they do not. One of the fascinating things about tension is the way in which its effects vary so widely. A challenge or conflict that turns out to be the stimulus that is the making of one person may spell doom, disaster, and breakdown to another. In general, response to tension depends on both its intensity and its duration, and on the personality and outlook of the person concerned.

What happens if a person is subjected to more tension than he or she can cope with?

If the tension proves to be too much for the person's coping mechanisms, some form of breakdown is inevitable. This may be social, psychiatric, or physical, and may in some way lead to high blood pressure, peptic ulcer, heart attack, depression, or addiction.

When does everyday tension cause medical problems?

Simply, when there is more of it than an individual can cope with. Tension or arousal is intended to lead to, and have its natural outlet in, some form of action. If that does not happen, perhaps because the action is blocked in some way, or because the amount of tension is greater than the opportunity for activities in which it can be either utilized or worked off, then it will build up, like steam in a pan, until the lid blows off. This may result in something as serious as a coronary thrombosis, stroke, or suicide. Yet the solution can be simple: a full recovery can be made by resting and changing to a more relaxed attitude. Otherwise, a vicious cycle can develop in which, as the ability to cope with tension becomes inadequate, the person pushes him- or herself harder to try to achieve results that he or she cannot attain. Often the person most in need of taking a rest, the workaholic, finds it hardest to slow down and take a calm look at the problems facing him or her.

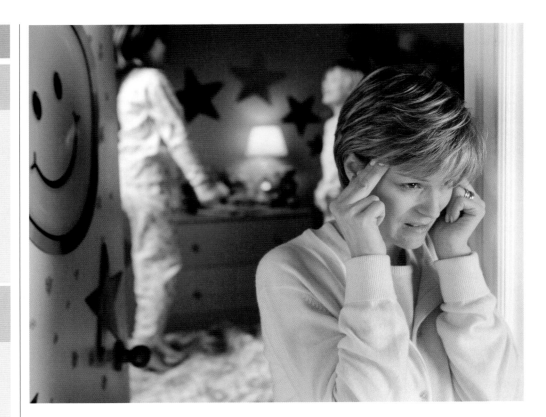

▲ *Often the apparently simple events of daily life, especially within the close environment of a family, can lead to excessive buildup of tension from which it is hard to find relief.*

interests. It may be total or partial, with an element of compromise. For instance, most members of the community agree to, or submit easily to, the rules of the herd and never get into any trouble, but some are always at odds and in difficulties with it. Generally, however, it is those who do not submit easily who are responsible for new ideas and progress. These people are driven by tension to experiment and explore new possibilities.

Reactions to tension

In all these reactions to tension there are three classes of response: those that a person can accept as normal; those that seem excessive or exaggerated; and those that are definitely not normal and represent some form of psychiatric illness. The difference between them, however, is really only one of degree. The response that occurs depends partly on the importance and intensity of the conflict and partly on the personality and mentality of the person concerned (see Personality). Therefore, it is not regarded as abnormal for people generally to submit to the conventions of their community with regard to acceptable behavior. However, persistent feelings of inferiority, unworthiness, groveling, and guilt over small matters are considered inappropriately excessive. However, manifestations of persistent depression, prolonged melancholy, and feelings of persecution are viewed as being definitely abnormal (see Depression). In the realm of escape as a response to tension, people regard jokes, hobbies, vacations, and fantasy as in plays and films as acceptable; they find heavy drinking, drug taking, and outbursts of temperamental behavior excessive; and they consider alcoholism, permanent running away, and suicide attempts as definitely abnormal (see Alcoholism; Suicide). The kinds of situation that are most likely to give rise to abnormal tension in people's lives today may be quite different from the more basic and immediate threats of hunger, thirst, cold, lack of shelter, fighting for food, and rivalry for partners to mate with that were the prime sources of emotional and physical conflict in the time of people's ancestors. However, 21st-century tensions operate and affect people in much the same way, and people need to be able to cope with them no less effectively to survive.

> See also: Coronary arteries and thrombosis; Family relationships; Psychiatry; Relaxation; Stress; Stress management; Wellness

Testes

The testes are the twin organs that control male fertility and the production of the sex hormone testosterone. These functions are so important that prompt treatment of any problems is essential.

The normal human male has two testes that develop in the embryo from a ridge of tissue at the back of the abdomen. When the testes have formed, they gradually move down inside the abdomen so that, at the time of birth, each testis has arrived in its final position, usually within the scrotum.

Function and structure

The function of the testes is twofold. First, they provide the site where sperm is manufactured; each sperm contains all the genetic information for that particular male. Second, the testes contain cells that produce the male sex hormone testosterone (see Testosterone), and

STRUCTURE OF THE TESTES

The testes consist of seminiferous tubules, where sperm are made; and interstitial cells, which produce the male hormone testosterone. Sperm is stored in the epididymis before passing along the vas deferens to be ejaculated.

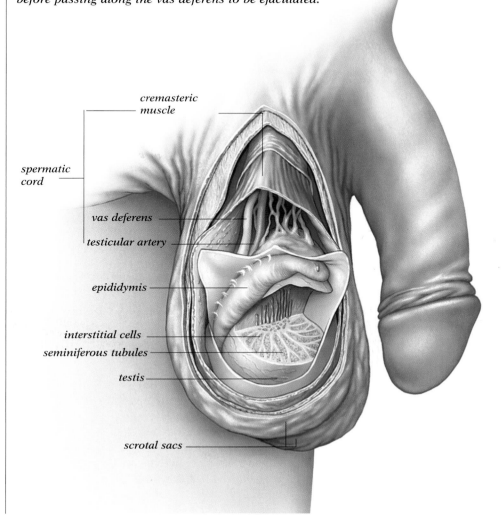

cremasteric muscle

spermatic cord

vas deferens

testicular artery

epididymis

interstitial cells

seminiferous tubules

testis

scrotal sacs

Questions and Answers

Does damage to the testes cause changes in secondary sex characteristics, such as facial hair or voice?

If insufficient male hormone is produced by the testes at puberty, the secondary sex characteristics, such as facial hair and a deep voice, fail to develop. This results in what is known as eunuchism. Once the voice has deepened, then removal of, or damage to, the testes will have no effect, but there will be a loss of sexual drive if the testes are removed in adulthood. Male hormones can be administered by injection.

My two-year-old appears to have only one testis in his scrotum. Will the other one appear at puberty?

It depends. You should see your doctor. If the testis is retractile, that is, it has been pulled up into the groin by an overactive muscle, then it will come down at puberty. If, however, it never reached the scrotum, then he will need a small operation in a year or two to bring it down.

One of my husband's testes has become larger than the other. There is no pain. Should he have it checked?

Yes. It is very important that he is seen by a doctor right away. The enlargement could be caused by a collection of fluid around the testis, or by a small tumor inside the testis. It should be apparent to a doctor which of these it is. If it is a tumor, there is a good chance that it can be cured.

Is it possible to get an infection in the testis that makes it tender and swollen?

Yes, but this is quite unusual in young men, and tenderness and swelling would be more likely to be caused by a twisting of the testis on the spermatic cord, cutting off its blood supply. These symptoms may also arise as a result of an STD, usually with chlamydia.

CONNECTION OF TESTIS WITH PENIS

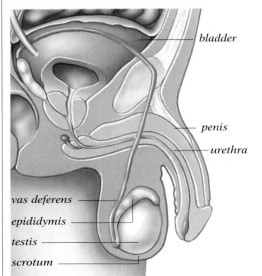

bladder

penis

urethra

vas deferens

epididymis

testis

scrotum

HYDROCELE

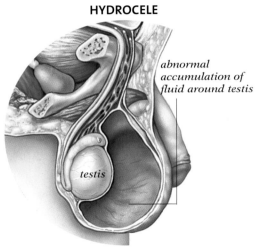

abnormal accumulation of fluid around testis

testis

▲ *An abnormal accumulation of fluid around the testes is a disorder called hydrocele.*

consequently, masculine characteristics, such as a deep voice, male hair distribution, and typical distribution of fat. These two functions are carried out by separate sets of cells within each of the testes; one function can fail without the other one necessarily doing so.

The testes are ovoid structures. Attached to the posterior of each one is a smaller structure shaped like a long comma. This is called the epididymis. The epididymis consists of a series of microscopically tiny tubes that collect sperm from the testis. These tubes connect together to form one tube, called the vas deferens, which transfers the sperm toward the base of the bladder. All these structures, with the exception of the vas deferens, are microscopic in size.

Each testis is suspended in the scrotum by a spermatic cord, which consists of the vas deferens, the testicular artery, and the testicular vein. The spermatic cord is surrounded by a tube of muscle called the cremasteric muscle. The spermatic cord, therefore, serves two purposes: first, to provide a blood supply to the testis; and second, to conduct sperm away from the testis.

What can go wrong?

For the vast majority of males, the testes carry out their complex functions without any problems. Sometimes, however, structural or functional difficulties do occur which can usually be successfully treated.

Undescended testes: In order for sperm to be manufactured, the testes have to be at a slightly lower temperature than the normal body temperature. For this reason the testes are suspended outside the abdominal cavity, in the scrotum.

At birth, however, it may be noticed that one testis has not descended into the scrotum. An undescended testis can have several effects: it will be unable to produce sperm; it may be damaged in the groin and be more prone to twisting, or torsion; and there is a slightly increased risk of developing a tumor. It is important to distinguish between an undescended testis and one that is retractile. The latter term means that the cremasteric muscle is overactive and has pulled the testis up into the groin. A retractile testis will probably descend into the scrotum at puberty; an undescended testis will not descend, and will require surgery. If the testis has not descended by the age of one, treatment is required. Sometimes a nasal spray is prescribed that stimulates the production of sex hormones which help to bring the testis into the scrotum, or a hormone may be injected into a muscle.

If these measures fail surgery is usually performed at the age of two or three. The operation for an undescended testis is called an orchiopexy. It consists of a small incision in the groin to find the testis, followed by stitching it into place in the scrotum. There is some evidence that if the operation is delayed beyond this age, irreversible damage to the testis may occur. However, even if a testis does not produce sperm because it has not descended, it still may be able to produce normal amounts of testosterone. One testis that is functioning normally should be perfectly adequate to produce sufficient sperm and testosterone (see Sperm).

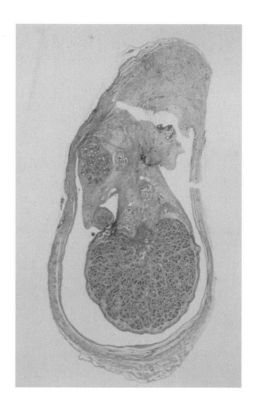

▲ *This cross section of the testes clearly shows the scrotum, the epididymis, the vas deferens, and the seminiferous tubules.*

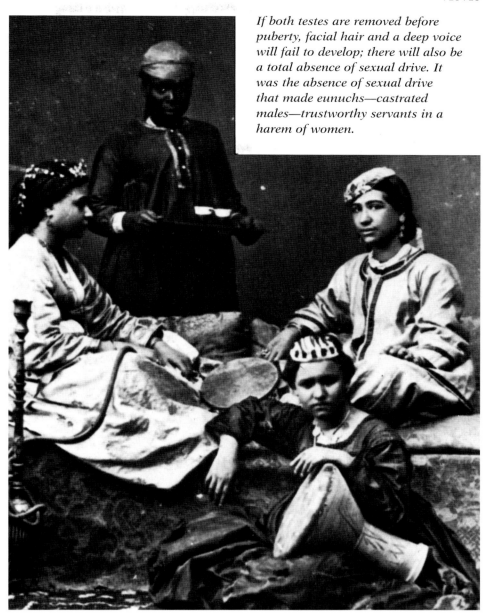

If both testes are removed before puberty, facial hair and a deep voice will fail to develop; there will also be a total absence of sexual drive. It was the absence of sexual drive that made eunuchs—castrated males—trustworthy servants in a harem of women.

Torsion: Some men have an abnormality in the way in which the testis hangs in the scrotum. This abnormality is present at birth, and usually affects both testes. The abnormality causes one of the testes to twist on its spermatic cord, leading to a sudden cutting off of the blood supply to the testis. The most common age for this to occur is the teens, but it can also happen in younger children or young adults.

The usual symptom of a torsion of the testis is extreme tenderness and the sudden onset of severe pain on one side of the scrotum. Untreated, the twisted testis swells and becomes inflamed, and eventually becomes gangrenous. Irreversible gangrene can occur within hours of the onset of the pain. Because of the swelling and inflammation, there is a danger that a case of torsion could be mistaken for infection. Infection in the testis in a teenager is rare, and all cases of inflammation of the testis in this age group should be treated as torsion until proved otherwise.

Treatment involves surgical exploration, untwisting of the testis, and fixing it with stitches so that it cannot twist again. If it is gangrenous, it will have to be removed. Because the abnormality is present on both sides, a small operation is usually done on the other side to prevent torsion from occurring.

Infection and inflammation: Sometimes infection can pass from the bladder along the vas deferens, and then gain access to the epididymis. This infection, called epididymitis, usually occurs in older men and may be a sexually acquired chlamydial infection. The symptoms are pain and swelling in one side of the scrotum. Usually the urine is infected and, after treatment with an appropriate antibiotic, the infection clears up. There are normally no long-term effects, but the patient may be prone to repeated attacks. Inflammation of the testis itself is known as orchitis. Infection with the mumps virus can cause orchitis and, if both testes are affected, can lead to sterility (see Mumps). Fortunately, however, this type of complication is rare.

Cysts: There are several different types of cyst that can occur in the testes. They are usually associated with some congenital abnormality, but may not become apparent until the patient is quite old. The first type is known as an epididymal cyst and shows itself as a lump attached to the testis; the testis can still be felt as a separate entity. Shining a strong light through the lump confirms that it is not solid, but is full of clear fluid.

The second type of cystic swelling is known as a hydrocele. This may be larger and is different from an epididymal cyst in that the fluid-filled cavity surrounds the testis so that the testis cannot be

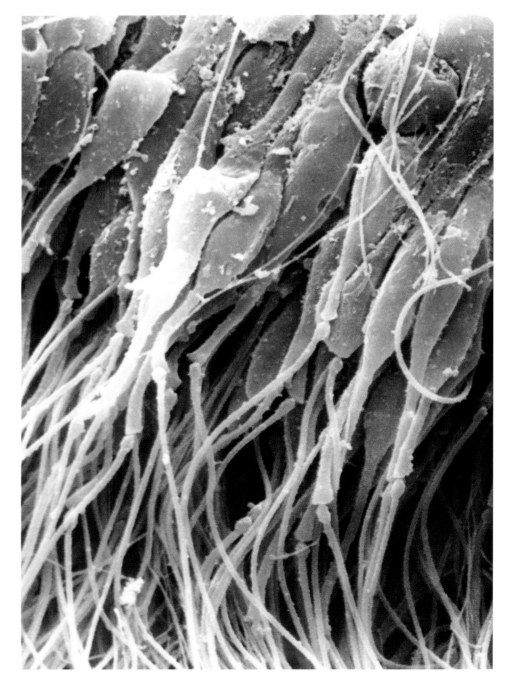

▲ *This image, taken using a scanning electron microscope and artificially colored, shows almost mature sperm embedded in the wall of a seminiferous tubule.*

are significant because they can cause a rise in the temperature of the tissues in the scrotum. This can lead to impairment of sperm production and infertility.

Treatment involves surgical removal of the large veins, and this sometimes leads to a rise in the sperm count.

Tumors of the testis

Tumors of the testis are actually quite rare in comparison with the incidence of some other tumors. Many of them can be cured completely, even though they are, technically speaking, a form of cancer. Testicular tumors generally occur in young men, between the ages of 18 and 40 years, although they can occur in other age groups.

The most common way in which they become apparent is that the patient notices that one testis is bigger than the other or irregular. There may not be any pain, but occasionally there is some tenderness.

Treatment involves removing the testis, followed by further investigations to see whether the tumor has spread. Even if it has spread, the results of treatment with X rays and special drugs are good.

Infertility

Infertility can be caused by many factors, but the fault may lie in the failure of the man to produce adequate sperm in the semen. There may be many reasons for this. First, there may be a blockage in the vas deferens so that the normal number of sperm produced in the testis cannot pass into the urethra during intercourse. Second, the testes may be failing to produce sperm, a condition that is possibly associated with a lack of testosterone. The failure of sperm production may be inherent in the testes, or it may be caused by other factors, such as general illness, cigarette smoking, increased heat in the testis caused by wearing underpants that are too tight and push the testes up into the groin, or the presence of a varicocele, which raises the temperature of the testes.

felt separately. The former type of cyst is entirely harmless. The second type is usually harmless but occasionally may be associated with underlying inflammation in the testis or, more rarely, a tumor.

The treatment of these cysts is to remove them surgically, but only if they are causing symptoms (see Cyst).

Varicocele: This is a condition in which the veins in the spermatic cord become enlarged and twisted, like varicose veins. The patient usually notices an aching sensation in the scrotum and may feel a lump just above the testis when he stands up. Because the lump is in fact the veins full of blood, it goes away when the patient lies down. Apart from causing a dragging, aching sensation, varicoceles

Various measures can be taken to increase the sperm count, such as wearing loose pants, taking regular cold scrotal douches, and maintaining good health. Hormone tablets may be prescribed. If there is a complete absence of sperm, and a blockage is suspected, surgery may be undertaken to bypass the blockage. This will be performed after a biopsy of the testes has shown normal production of sperm.

See also: **Biopsy; Infertility; Intercourse; Sex; Sexual dysfunction; Sexually transmitted diseases; Surgery; Tumors; Urethra**

Testosterone

Testosterone is the most important of the male sex hormones, and it is responsible for producing typical male characteristics: a deep voice, beard growth, and increase in muscle bulk.

The glands of the body produce many different hormones—substances that act as chemical messengers. They are made and released in one part of the body and then travel (mainly in the blood) to other body cells where they bring about their effects.

One important group of hormones is the sex hormones. These are different in men and women, and they are responsible for controlling fertility and reproduction, and for producing distinctive physical characteristics, such as deep voice, beard growth, and increased muscle bulk in men, and breast growth in women.

The male sex hormones are called androgens, and the most important of the androgens is testosterone. Like all the sex hormones it is a steroid hormone; it is known as an anabolic steroid (see Steroids).

How is testosterone produced?

Testosterone is produced in specialized cells (called Leydig cells) in the testes (see Testes). It is also produced in very small amounts in the ovaries of women.

Testosterone production begins when a boy reaches puberty (see Adolescence). A hormone called luteinizing hormone (LH) is secreted by the pituitary. LH is then carried in the blood to the testes, where it stimulates the Leydig cells to secrete testosterone. During puberty, LH, and therefore testosterone, is secreted only at night; but later, as LH levels rise during the day, testosterone is secreted 24 hours a day.

In women, testosterone secreted by the ovaries is converted into a hormone called estradiol, which plays an important role in ovulation and in the menstrual cycle.

What does testosterone do?

The most noticeable effects of testosterone occur at puberty, when it is responsible for many of the physical changes of maturation that take place. During puberty, there are changes in both the external and the internal genitalia. The penis increases in length and width (see Penis and Disorders), and the scrotum becomes pigmented. Internally, the seminal vesicles, which lie just behind the bladder, and the prostate gland, which is tiny at birth, start to enlarge. The prostate increases to about the size of a walnut. They both begin to secrete seminal fluid.

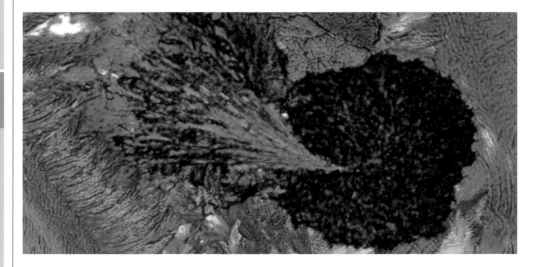

▲ *A colored and magnified (x260) photomicrograph of the male hormone testosterone.*

Testosterone causes the larynx to enlarge and the vocal cords to increase in length and thickness. These changes cause a boy's voice to break and become deeper. At around the same time a beard begins to appear, with a growth of chest, underarm, and pubic hair. The amount of body hair also increases over the whole body. All androgens have what is called an anabolic effect, that is, they raise the rate of protein synthesis and lower the rate at which protein is broken down. The effect is to increase muscle bulk, especially in the chest and shoulders, and to accelerate growth of the long bones (in the arms and legs), especially during early puberty. When puberty is finished, testosterone stops the growth of the long bones by ossifying the cartilage plates (epiphyses) at the end of the bones.

The skin changes that often occur in adolescence are also caused by androgens. Androgens stimulate the sebaceous glands in the skin to secrete sebum. If the glands secrete too much sebum, this can lead to acne (see Acne and Pimples).

Around this time the sex drive begins to increase, and boys start to show an interest in girls, and also to produce sperm. Ejaculation sometimes occurs during the night. Testosterone also promotes a more aggressive attitude, which is a characteristically male trait. The testes will produce testosterone throughout a man's life. After puberty, testosterone maintains the male sex characteristics, and with a hormone called follicle-stimulating hormone (FSH) it is involved in the production of sperm in the seminiferous tubules of the testes. Hereditary baldness in men is also linked to testosterone (see Baldness).

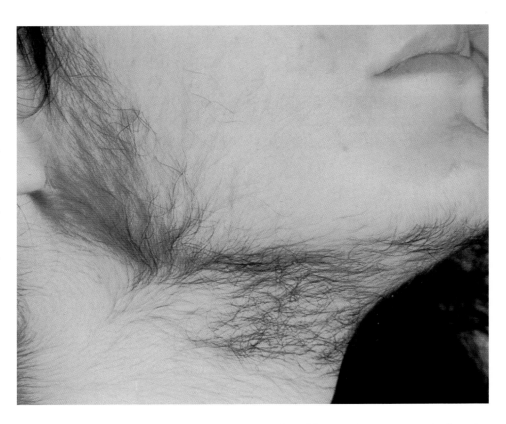

▲ *This young woman has developed excessive facial hair or hirsutism. It is thought to be associated with a hormonal disturbance producing excess testosterone.*

What can go wrong?

Excess testosterone, either secreted by the body or taken as a drug, causes problems in both males and females. In women, overproduction of testosterone causes the development of masculine features such as an increase in facial hair and body hair, deepening of the voice, and some hair loss. Facial spots may develop and testosterone can also lead to an increase in body weight. It is very rare for a woman to produce an excess of testosterone, but occasionally it may be the result of an androgen-secreting ovarian tumor, or an ovarian cyst.

In adult males the presence of excess testosterone accentuates male physical characteristics. It can also cause a condition called priapism, which is a painful persistent erection. It may be the result of a testicular tumor. Excess testosterone given to stimulate puberty may interfere with normal growth or cause over-rapid sexual development. Initially the testosterone increases bone growth but adult height is reduced because the testosterone causes the long bones to stop growing too soon.

A deficiency of testosterone is far more common than an excess of the hormone. A deficiency may occur if the testes are diseased, or if the pituitary gland does not secrete LH. The effects vary, depending on whether the deficiency develops before or after puberty. If it develops before puberty the boy's limbs continue to grow so that his final adult height will be increased, and he will have particularly long arms and legs. Other typical effects include decreased body hair and beard growth, smooth skin, a high-pitched voice, reduced sexual drive and performance, underdevelopment of the genitalia, and poor muscle development. Teenage boys with delayed puberty are usually treated with testosterone. This boosts puberty artificially, and so avoids psychological problems (see Puberty). Testosterone may also be given to men who have become infertile because of a deficiency of pituitary hormones.

Treatment

Testosterone can be given as a pellet implanted under the skin of the abdominal wall under local anesthesia or as an injection into the muscle, or it can be taken orally. All forms of treatment are effective and safe. Occasionally, if testosterone is given to an adult who has never been through puberty, testosterone can trigger aggression.

Menopausal women are sometimes given implants of testosterone in addition to other types of hormones. In the condition female transsexualism, the individuals have the appearance of femininity, but believe that they belong to the male sex. After discussions of their condition with a doctor and psychiatrist, it may be decided that the best solution is for the transsexual to take regular doses of testosterone. This gradually deepens the voice, promotes hair growth on the face and chest, decreases feminine fat, and gives an appearance of maleness.

See also: **Hormones; Ovaries**

Tetanus

Can I be immunized against tetanus?

Yes, you can and definitely should be. Children are given a vaccine against this serious disease with their first series of injections and are given a booster dose as they start school. Older people may not have been vaccinated and should ask their doctor for the immunization to avoid a risk of infection. If you have been vaccinated you should have a booster dose every 10 years. When people go to the emergency room with wounds, they are usually given a booster. The vaccination is against the toxin rather than the bacteria that make it, since it is the toxin that causes all the trouble.

Is tetanus in a wound made by a rusty, rather than a clean, object?

No. Tetanus spores are very common in our environment, and it is possible to infect yourself, even with an object that appears clean. However, the highest concentration of spores is found in soil and in manure. An object like a rusty nail is perhaps more likely to have been in contact with spores; therefore you may be more likely to get an infection from such an object.

Does tetanus cause paralysis so that you can hear but can't move or speak?

No. Tetanus is caused by a toxin that acts directly on the nervous system. The effects of the toxin are to produce muscle rigidity, leading to lockjaw, a name sometimes given to the disease, and to produce spasms. The spasms can be exhausting and even fatal if they occur frequently. To prevent them, sedation is used. If this fails, the patient may be deliberately paralyzed with drugs and put on a respirator.

A rusty nail, a clumsy step, and the resulting wound could be the ideal breeding ground for the virulent bacterium that causes tetanus. The disease can be fatal, so adequate immunization is of the utmost importance.

Tetanus is a frightening and dangerous disease that can be fatal, even with the best medical care. However, all the techniques of intensive care can be brought to bear on sufferers in developed countries, and there is no doubt that modern treatment does significantly reduce the number of deaths from this disease.

Cause

Tetanus is caused by a bacterium called *Clostridium tetani*. The organism is found freely in soil, and is even more common in manured and cultivated soil, since it is very common in animal dung. However, the organism is not confined to soil; street dust from the center of a town certainly contains the spores of the bacteria, and spores can even be found inside buildings in large amounts (see Bacteria).

The bacterium has one very important characteristic that controls the way the disease behaves; it is killed by oxygen and grows only in oxygen-free surroundings. That is why the bacteria have to be introduced into the body through a wound, such as a cut, since the blood supply, and therefore the oxygen supply, is cut off as a result of the tissue damage. The deeper and more contaminated a wound, the higher the risk of tetanus (see Wounds).

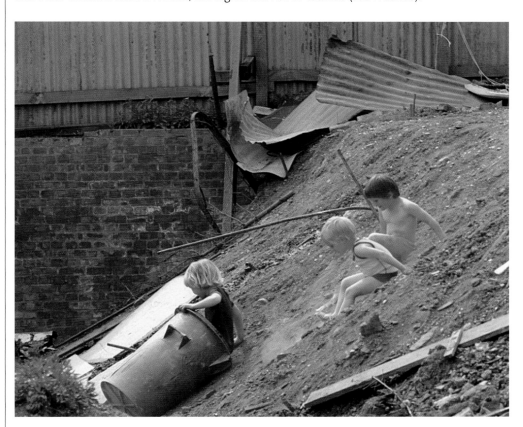

▲ *It is not uncommon for tetanus to be picked up in cities. The bacterium makes spores that are resistant to the effects of drying and heat, and can survive for long periods in dust. These children, if not immunized, would therefore be at risk, simply because they are playing in a dusty area where they are exposed to injury.*

The toxin made by the bacterium is a deadly substance, exceeded in potency only by the toxin responsible for botulism. Only one-tenth of a milligram is a fatal dose for an adult. The toxin is produced in the site of a wound that has been contaminated by the bacterium; from there, the toxin passes into the spinal cord and the brain. It is thought that it travels through the nerves, although transmission in the bloodstream could also be important. Once in the nervous system the toxin cannot be neutralized by antibodies, either produced by the body after immunization or given as antitoxin (see Nervous System).

Symptoms

The incubation period is six to 10 days as a rule, although in rare cases it may be several months. In some cases, symptoms can occur extremely quickly, in 24 hours.

There is a short vague illness with headache, general illness, and fever, but the important first signs are due to the generalized muscle rigidity that is one of the two classic symptoms of the disease. This especially affects the jaw muscles—giving rise to lockjaw, by which name the disease is sometimes known—the muscles of the abdomen, which are found to be rigid on examination, and the muscles of the back. Eventually, the back may be arched over and the neck bent back.

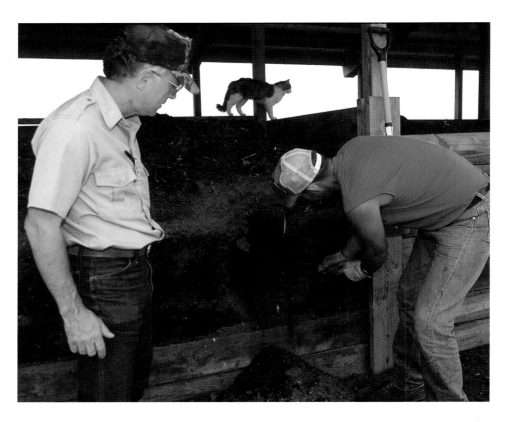

▲ *People who work on the land—such as gardeners and farmers—are most likely to catch tetanus. The bacterium is commonly found in animal dung, a normal component of fertilized and cultivated soil.*

Spasms develop later and can be brought on by any stimulus. Minor spasms may simply affect the face, with contraction of the facial muscles into a ghastly grin, known by the chilling Latin title *risus sardonicus*, meaning sardonic smile. Breathing can be affected by these spasms and when they become more generalized they lead to even more exaggerated arching of the back and neck.

The difficulty in caring for tetanus patients really becomes marked when the disease interferes with the way that the brain controls vital functions. The heart may be affected, leading to abnormalities of rhythm and either very low or very high blood pressure. Sometimes the temperature may increase very rapidly.

Treatment

The aim of treatment is to maintain the patient over the period of his or her illness and prevent a possibly fatal outcome from occurring. Problems that can occur include exhaustion due to spasm, asphyxia during spasm, pneumonia due to stomach contents entering the lungs, and death due to disorders of control of vital functions, such as the heartbeat and blood pressure.

In milder cases, simple sedation and the avoidance of all types of disturbance will

▲ *Once in the body, the bacterium may grow in an area with no blood supply, making it difficult for antibiotics to reach.*

prevent spasms, but in the more severe cases a tracheotomy is performed to make an opening in the windpipe (tracheostomy), and the patient is totally paralyzed using curare (a paralyzing drug), while breathing is taken over by a respirator. The disease is likely to be most severe when the incubation period has been short and when there has been less than 48 hours between the first symptom and the first spasm.

Prevention

Immunization with tetanus toxoid is given with a baby's first immunization, and boosters are given when children start school and on leaving. After that, a booster should be given every 10 years—or more often if you are at special risk, for example, if you work on the land. In people who have not been immunized it is necessary to give an antitoxin after any serious wound (see Immunization).

The risk of contracting tetanus can be reduced by immediately cleansing all wounds, even minor wounds, and the use of large doses of penicillin. Adequate immunization, however, is the best option, as it can eliminate the risk completely.

See also: **Botulism; Tracheostomy**

Tetracyclines

The tetracycline group provides important weapons in the doctor's armory of antibiotic drugs. Tetracyclines are used against a range of diseases and infections—but judiciously, since resistance to tetracyclines can develop.

Questions and Answers

I am allergic to penicillin. Does this mean that I am also allergic to tetracyclines?

No. In fact, the tetracycline group of antibiotics could be very valuable to you simply because you are allergic to the penicillins. They are effective and safe against a wide range of common infections.

My doctor often gives me a tetracycline for bronchitis. When I was pregnant, however, she no longer prescribed it. Why was this?

A tetracycline shouldn't be used in pregnancy, since it forms a deposit in the baby's teeth and stains them. The same thing happens to a lesser extent in the baby's bones. Tetracyclines can form deposits in the teeth at any age up to about eight or nine, so they are generally not given to children whose teeth are still growing.

My daughter is a nurse, and she tells me that many bacteria are now resistant to tetracyclines. Does this mean that they are no longer useful as antibiotics?

Your daughter probably works in a hospital where tetracyclines are not often used. Resistance can develop to tetracyclines, and in a hospital the resistant bacteria can be easily passed from patient to patient. Yet some types of infection will respond only to tetracyclines, like typhus, psittacosis, and brucellosis.

My doctor gave me tetracycline and I got severe diarrhea. Am I allergic to this particular drug?

No, people often get diarrhea as a result of treatment with any antibiotic because the antibiotic not only kills off the bacteria that are causing trouble, but also kills bacteria that normally live in the colon. This leads to a disturbance in its function, and diarrhea results.

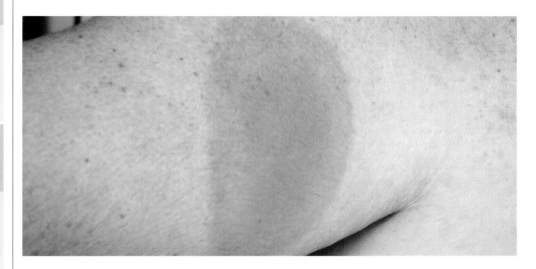

▲ *Tetracyclines are used to treat Lyme disease, which is caused by a tick bite. The disease causes a large red rash around the insect's bite, as seen on this man's arm.*

Tetracyclines are used to treat a number of common diseases caused by bacteria and provide one of the only effective forms of treatment for many less common infections. Tetracyclines work by blocking the action of the ribosomes (the cell's protein factory) within the bacteria. Although treatment with tetracyclines will stop a bacterium from growing, the drugs may not succeed in killing it off. For this reason, tetracyclines are called bacteriostatic drugs (drugs that stop bacteria) as opposed to the bactericidal drugs such as penicillin, which actually kill off individual bacteria.

Effectiveness

Tetracyclines are effective against a wide range of organisms, including those responsible for acne, Lyme disease, cholera, chlamydial infections (such as psittacosis), typhus, and Rocky Mountain spotted fever (see Cholera; Lyme Disease; Rocky Mountain Spotted Fever; Typhus).

However, one problem that has occurred since their introduction in the 1950s is that a number of the common organisms causing infection have become resistant to the effects of tetracyclines. This is a problem that occurs with many antibiotics, but it seems to be particularly severe with tetracyclines. Because there is a certain amount of resistance to these drugs, they are used less in hospitals, where resistant strains of bacteria would have the opportunity to spread from patient to patient. There is much less chance that a patient attending his or her doctor's office would have caught a resistant bacterium, so tetracylines remain safe and effective for people who are normally fit and who are removed from the risk of catching hospital infections.

Dangers

Side effects may include vomiting, diarrhea, nausea, and, rarely, rash and itching. However, the main danger is that tetracyclines tend to get bound into growing bones and teeth. While there is little adverse effect on the bones, the teeth may become stained with defective enamel. Therefore, children whose teeth are still growing and pregnant mothers should avoid tetracyclines (see Teeth and Teething).

> See also: Antibiotics; Bacteria; Infection and infectious diseases; Psittacosis; Side effects

Thalassemia

Thalassemia is a blood disease and is one of the most common inherited diseases—especially in Mediterranean regions. Although it can be fatal in its most severe form, blood transfusions can improve life expectancy.

Thalassemia is a form of anemia, and it results from abnormalities in the structure of hemoglobin, the oxygen-carrying component of blood.

There are two basic forms of the disease: thalassemia major and thalassemia minor. In the minor form, there are usually no serious ill effects, but the major form is often fatal (see Anemia).

Causes

Hemoglobin is responsible for carrying oxygen from the lungs to the body tissues. It is made up of two substances that are chemically bound together; "heme," the iron-containing central core of a hemoglobin molecule; and "globin," the protein constituent that exists as a chain. The body produces a number of different globin chains, but it is the alpha and beta chains that determine the thalassemic condition. Each molecule of hemoglobin has four globin chains attached to its central portion. Normal hemoglobin in an adult, called hemoglobin A, is made from two alpha and two beta chains. The construction of the chain is determined by inherited genes (see Genetics; Heredity).

If the normal construction of the globin chains fails and insufficient amounts are produced of either the alpha or the beta chains, the formation of hemoglobin is affected and thalassemia is the result. The failure can be caused by both the presence of an abnormal gene and an abnormality in what is called the transcription process: that is, converting the genetic instructions into the production of new protein molecules.

Beta thalassemia

People inherit two genes from their parents that control the production of beta chains. If one of the genes is faulty, the outcome is beta thalassemia minor, a form of thalassemia that gives no serious trouble. However, when both genes are defective, then the very serious beta thalassemia

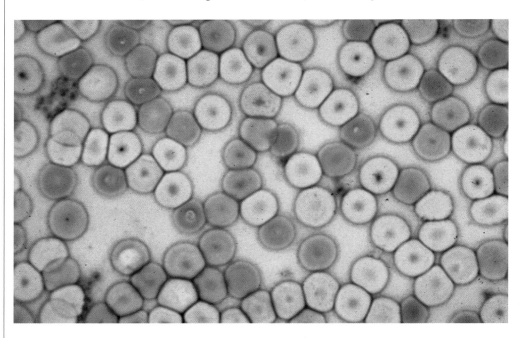

▲ *In thalassemia, the body tries to compensate for the lack of hemoglobin in the red blood cells by producing extra red cells, as shown above.*

THALASSEMIA AND MALARIA: ARE THEY CONNECTED?

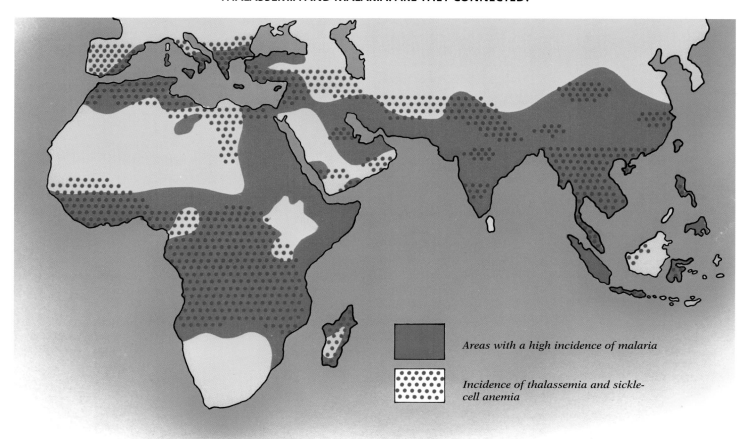

Areas with a high incidence of malaria

Incidence of thalassemia and sickle-cell anemia

major is the result. In this disease, the faulty hemoglobin, called hemoglobin F, which is normally found only in the fetus, is very slow to give up the oxygen to the tissues, and this leads to overstimulation of the bone marrow. The marrow expands and may deform the bones that contain it (see Marrow and Transplants). This long-standing and serious anemic condition is particularly dangerous for children because it restricts their growth.

Alpha thalassemia
Alpha thalassemia is slightly more complex, but not as serious, owing to the fact that everyone inherits four genes that are responsible for the production of alpha globin chains. If one or two of these genes are defective in any way, then the result is alpha thalassemia minor, which is not serious; the sufferer has only slight anemia, but will need treatment. When there are three defective alpha genes, this produces a type of hemoglobin called hemoglobin H, which results in hemoglobin H disease. Red blood cells break down easily, and this leads to anemia and jaundice. Although this condition cannot be cured, it can be successfully controlled through blood transfusions, and the sufferer can lead a nearly normal life (see Blood; Blood Transfusion). However, when all four alpha chain genes are missing, a type of blood is produced that is not compatible with life and the fetus either aborts or is stillborn.

Treatment
The treatment for the different types of thalassemia is similar; patients are provided with regular blood transfusions to keep the

▲ *Thalassemia and sickle-cell anemia are particularly common in certain areas of the world and, significantly, these are areas where malaria thrives. It is possible that genetic mutations that cause these blood diseases have an important side effect, and that they may offer some form of protection against malaria.*

level of hemoglobin high; this maintains the supply of oxygen to the tissues. The regularity of blood transfusions depends on the type and severity of the anemia. Since frequent blood transfusions can result in a dangerous buildup of iron, some patients may need daily treatment with a special drug that allows the kidneys to exrete excess iron safely in the urine. Treatment may also include antibiotics to counter infection, and somtimes the spleen is removed.

Prevention
Genetic counseling is the only preventive measure that can be taken. Using simple tests, it is possible to determine whether two people have the genes for beta thalassemia. When this is found, one in four of the children is expected to have beta thalassemia major.

It is possible to analyze the blood of the fetus at about 20 weeks into the pregnancy to see if there are any beta chains being produced. If this is not the case, then a baby considered at risk is likely to have the disease, and it may be best to terminate the pregnancy.

See also: **Genetic diseases and disorders; Screening**

Thalidomide

What is thalidomide and where did it come from?

Thalidomide is the generic name for a hypnotic (sleep-inducer) drug marketed under a total of 51 trade names, including Asmaval, Distaval, Kevadon, Contergan, Tensival, and Valgraine. The drug is composed of carbon, nitrogen, oxygen, and hydrogen. It was invented and developed in West Germany by the Chemie Grünenthal company and was sold in 46 countries.

The inventor of thalidomide, Wilhelm Kunz, was trying to find a more efficient peptide (one of the molecules that make up protein) for use in antibiotics. Thalidomide was not a great improvement on existing peptides, and might have been abandoned had not Herbert Keller, one of Kunz's colleagues, noticed that its molecular structure was similar to some sedatives.

Grünenthal's tests showed that it was an effective sedative, with no side effects and, incredibly, no toxic effect at any concentration. It was thought to be the first totally safe sleeping pill ever discovered, and its early success in Germany contributed to its acceptance elsewhere in the world.

Could a tragedy like thalidomide happen again?

In the wake of the thalidomide tragedy, many new controls were introduced to prevent any such recurrence, and drug companies now have much more sophisticated testing procedures than were available in the 1950s.

However, it is both economically and practically impossible for any drug to be declared totally safe. No amount of laboratory and animal tests can reliably predict the long-term effects of a drug on humans. Even human tests are inadequate, since people are very different from one another. It is less likely now that a drug as dangerous as thalidomide could be marketed, but it is not out of the question.

Thalidomide was once considered a wonder drug, but now the very name strikes a chill to the heart: thousands of babies suffered horrific deformities because their mothers took it in early pregnancy. What went wrong?

Thalidomide is a synthetic hypnotic drug composed of carbon, hydrogen, nitrogen, and oxygen (see Hypnotic Drugs). Its molecular structure is similar to that of some widely used and very effective sedatives such as glutethimide, although the similarity is slight (see Sedatives). In the late 1950s and early 1960s, sleeping pills formed an enormous part of the drug market in the United States and abroad. Thalidomide was the first apparently safe sleeping pill, and it sold by the million.

The "wonder drug"
Wilhelm Kunz, a chemist with Chemie Grünenthal in West Germany, invented thalidomide. His colleague Herbert Keller recognized the drug's sedative potential, and Grünenthal tested it for its efficacy and safety. There appeared to be no side effects and no maximum dose. The tests would later be questioned, but the company believed it had a wonder drug.

However, soon after the drug's introduction, some side effects were reported in adults. By the end of the first year, sales rose and Grünenthal dismissed the reports and made even stronger claims for thalidomide. A leaflet produced by the British distributors stated that "Distaval (thalidomide) can be given with complete safety to pregnant women and nursing mothers, without adverse effect on mother or child," even though no reproductive tests had been done.

Side effects
Adverse reports increased in number and confirmed that the drug caused peripheral neuritis: numbness in the extremities, cramps, pins and needles, weakness, and loss of motor control. Grünenthal continued to market the drug, and in May 1961 a thalidomide baby was born in Australia. It was badly malformed and died one week later, after unsuccessful emergency surgery. Within three weeks, two more such babies were born in the same hospital and the obstetrician

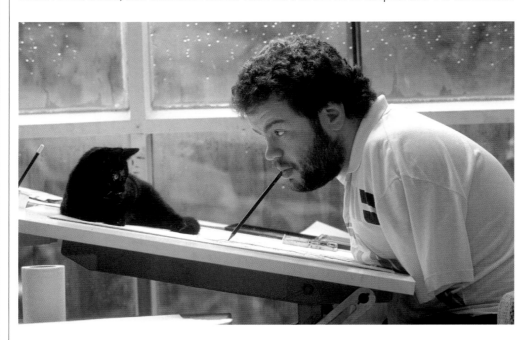

▲ *The artist Tom Yendell, who was affected by thalidomide, taught himself to draw and paint by holding pencils and brushes in his mouth instead of his hands. People with thalidomide deformities have found various ways to surmount their disabilities.*

Dr. William McBride set out to find the cause. He discovered a common factor. All three mothers had taken only one drug: thalidomide.

It was not until similar reports were made in Germany, and after pressure from the German press, that the company finally agreed to withdraw the drug in November 1961. Even so, governments were slow to respond and several hundred children were born malformed even after thalidomide's devastating effects were known.

A year after it was withdrawn in Europe, it was still available in Japan without prescription; the Swedish distributor continued to sell it in Argentina after it was banned in Sweden; in Italy it was still on sale, under 10 different trade names, 10 months after it had been withdrawn in Germany. The Food and Drug Administration banned the drug in the United States, and so spared much suffering.

The drug's effect on the unborn child was horrific and widespread. It is known that 50 to 80 percent of women who took the drug during the first trimester of pregnancy had deformed babies. Several babies were affected by a single dose. The first trimester of pregnancy is the crucial stage of fetal development when the limb buds form. Thalidomide arrested this growth and that of the internal organs.

Many of the children were born with such extensive deformities that they did not survive. Those that lived, about 7,500 worldwide, were sometimes badly deformed. Doctors and nurses were often unprepared to help the parents deal with the tragedy. This strain was made worse by the fact that at the time no one but a few doctors, and Grünenthal, suspected the cause, and parents blamed themselves and each other for their children's deformities.

Often nurses were unable to tell parents what the baby looked like, and kept them apart until they left the hospital. As a result, one mother discovered her child had no arms only after she got home. Failure to give parents adequate help, support, and guidance in accepting their handicapped children led to problems of rejection in some cases (see Handicaps). Society recoiled from the children, emotionally and financially; it was 10 years before financial settlements were made.

Could it have been foreseen?

Grünenthal claimed that it was not usual to test for reproductive effects, and that even if he had performed such tests they would

THE CRUCIAL STAGE OF FETAL DEVELOPMENT

During the second month of pregnancy, the fetal limb buds rapidly develop into fully formed limbs (below). Thalidomide arrested this development. Like most drugs, it was able to pass across the placenta by a simple process of diffusion.

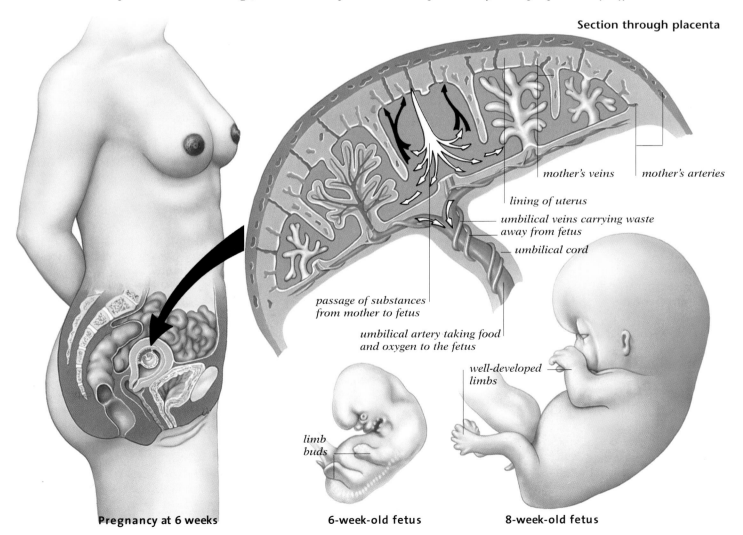

Section through placenta

mother's veins

mother's arteries

lining of uterus

umbilical veins carrying waste away from fetus

umbilical cord

passage of substances from mother to fetus

umbilical artery taking food and oxygen to the fetus

well-developed limbs

limb buds

Pregnancy at 6 weeks

6-week-old fetus

8-week-old fetus

have been carried out on rats, which do not show the effect. In many larger companies, however, it was already routine to test on pregnant animals. Several laboratories—including Distillers' Company (Biochemicals), the distributor of thalidomide in the UK—used rabbits, which do show the drug's teratogenic (deformity-causing) effects. It was known that drugs can cross the placental barrier and affect the unborn child, just as essential substances such as oxygen and nutrients do (see Placenta).

All of this, however, might have been excusably overlooked. What cannot be justified is that the drug was still being sold as safe for pregnant women long after it was known to cause serious neural side effects in adults (see Nervous System), and that, even after the birth defects were discovered in Japan, over a year elapsed before it was withdrawn from sale in that country.

Partly as a result of this tragedy, in 1970 new controls were effected, such as the formation of the Committee on the Safety of Medicines in the UK, and aids to the disabled were made available. Even the regulations and sophisticated techniques that now exist cannot guarantee that this tragedy will not recur. Since successes hugely outnumber tragedies, the balance is in the favor of nonrecurrence. However, just one mistake like thalidomide can have calamitous effects.

MOLECULAR STRUCTURE OF THALIDOMIDE

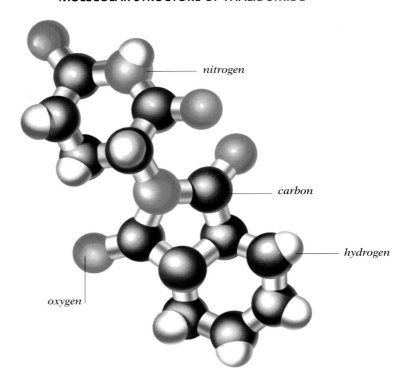

nitrogen

carbon

hydrogen

oxygen

▲ *Thalidomide was first developed as an artificial protein component, but it was found to have sedative properties, its structure being similar to that of other sedatives.*

The thalidomide story continues

As a result of the thalidomide disaster, most doctors and pharmacologists wanted to have nothing more to do with the drug. However, there remained a few researchers who realized that such a powerful drug was likely to have some useful applications.

In 1964, careful observations of patients with Hansen's disease (leprosy) who were taking thalidomide suggested that the drug might help certain phases of the disease (see Hansen's Disease). Many trials have since proved that this is, indeed, the case. Thalidomide has no direct effect on the leprosy bacillus, but it has a powerful effect on one of the types of acute flare-up reactions of the disease that can cause serious tissue destruction. The drug is effective in over 90 percent of cases and may bring about improvement within 24 hours. As a result, it has now been used by leprologists for years.

Graft-versus-host disease is a complication of bone marrow transplantation. It is a reaction of the transplanted cells against the tissues of the recipient, and it occurs in about 40 percent of patients who survive transplantation. However, it has a high mortality rate. Trials have shown that thalidomide is a safe and effective drug for this serious condition. The drug is not a complete cure, but has proved the most effective therapy to date. It has been shown to be effective in 20 percent of cases that resist treatment with antirejection drugs such as corticosteroids and cyclosporin (see Marrow and Transplants; Steroids).

A research paper in the prestigious *New England Journal of Medicine* for 22 May, 1997, reported that thalidomide had proved to be an effective treatment for the painful, debilitating, and persistent mouth ulcers that are a common feature of AIDS (see AIDS; Ulcers). In this trial, 55 percent of patients who received thalidomide had complete healing of their ulcers within four weeks. Only 7 percent of those who did not have thalidomide showed healing. Other trials have shown a cure rate as high as 81 percent. Thalidomide does not act against HIV, but may have a role in improving the general condition of people with AIDS.

Many other conditions have been shown to respond to, or to be helped by, thalidomide. These include various skin disorders caused by immune system malfunction; ulcerative colitis; rheumatoid arthritis; the genital and esophageal ulcers of Behçet's disease; and the severe and prolonged pain that often follows shingles, known as postherpetic neuralgia (see Colon and Colitis; Neuralgia; Rheumatoid Arthritis; Shingles).

The continuing thalidomide story is not all positive, however. The known effects on the early fetus make it imperative that the drug should not be used on women if there is any possibility of pregnancy. If there is no alternative, contraception must be 100 percent effective (see Contraception).

In addition, other side effects of thalidomide, especially on the nerves, appear to be potentially more serious than had at first been thought. Because of these dangers, thalidomide is a strictly controlled drug that is available only under prescribed conditions. As a result, exhaustive clinical guidelines for the use of thalidomide worldwide have been produced for doctors.

> **See also:** Birth defects; Congenital disorders; Fetus; Pharmacy

Therapy

What exactly does the word "therapy" mean?

"Therapy" is a general term and, although it is often used to mean psychotherapy, it should not be limited to any one group. A therapy is a treatment of any kind for a medical or psychological disorder. A medical dictionary usually contains 80 or more entries for procedures or techniques described as therapies.

Does the word "therapy" imply that the method actually works?

No, and people are often misled. The term should not be used unless there the method has proved to be effective. People who develop new therapies believe that they do work, but the care with which some of these are tested can be questionable.

If a therapy makes someone feel better, isn't that a sufficient justification for its use?

Up to a point. Scientific therapists make an important distinction between symptoms and the underlying disease process that causes them. Temporarily removing symptoms and making a person feel better can have serious consequences if it delays the start of conventional treatment that is rational and known to be completely effective.

Many people think that homeopathy works. Others think it illogical. Who is right?

Feeling better has nothing to do with reason. It may be that if a treatment is followed by an apparent recovery, this is attributed to the treatment, and will be remembered. The many occasions when the same treatment has had no effect are ignored and forgotten.

The term "therapy" covers a range of methods of treatment for physical and psychiatric disorders. Some have been scientifically proved to be effective; for other therapies, the evidence of their potential benefits is anecdotal.

Therapy is any form of treatment intended to relieve a disorder or disease of the body or mind. The word "therapy" is derived from the Greek word *therapeia*, meaning "attendance." Some therapies are based on ideas of which doctors are skeptical, but gradually the benefits of certain alternative and complementary therapies are becoming recognized.

Since therapy covers all forms of medical treatment, it includes the use of drugs to treat disease, which is called pharmacological therapeutics, and all forms of surgery. The choice of therapy clearly depends on the type of illness or injury that a patient is suffering from; the patient's personal choice and family circumstances are also taken into consideration.

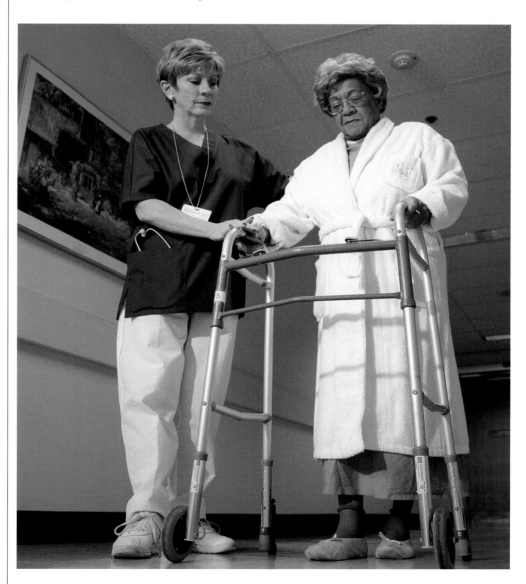

▲ *Physical therapy is a scientifically proved therapy that aims to restore a patient's full range of movement and mobility after an injury or surgery.*

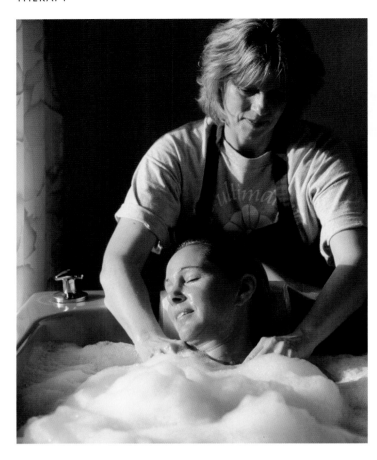

▲ *Water plays a role in more than one form of therapy. In hydrotherapy, patients lie in a warm bath or Jacuzzi, and physical therapy sessions may take place in water.*

Physical therapy

After a severe illness, injury, or surgery, many people are immobile and are left with muscles weakened through inactivity. Physical therapy aims to rehabilitate and to help people become more independent. Techniques are used that incorporate exercise to build up injured areas; massage can help to get stiff joints moving and improve and strengthen weak muscles (see Joints; Muscles).

Psychotherapies

These include therapies based on psychoanalysis, which are a range of psychoanalytic methods that aim to help people identify, face up to, and then work through their psychological problems. Psychotherapy can also involve families or groups as well as single people. These therapies are useful when the cause of the problem is not immediately apparent; the therapist tries to discover past events that have been instrumental in causing the person's present behavior and depression.

Behavior therapy is used to help change behavior, especially in people suffering from obsessive-compulsive disorder, phobias, and many forms of anxiety disorder. The therapy can involve desensitization, breathing techniques, and relaxation.

Complementary therapies

Although complementary therapies are still not completely understood, and some have not undergone rigorous testing, others

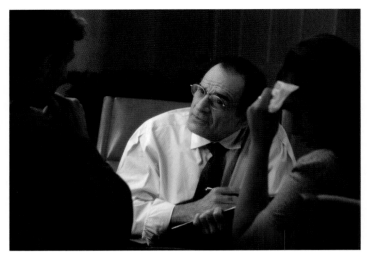

▲ *A psychotherapist interacts with his or her patients and encourages them to talk through their problems, rather than relying on drug treatment.*

have been used for centuries with considerable success. Certain complementary therapies have the approval of conventional medicine; and acupuncture and biofeedback are substantiated by scientific research. Acupuncture has been used to relieve many conditions and it is believed that the needles, when inserted into particular areas of the body, can release natural painkillers.

Chiropractic can be helpful in relieving pain in many people suffering from spinal disorders that cause neck and back pain. Although chiropractic is generally regarded as a safe practice, there is a small risk of complications such as spinal cord damage.

Some complementary therapies encourage valuable physical and mental habits and attitudes that can help to promote health. These include the Alexander technique, art therapy, biofeedback, dance movement therapy, hatha yoga (see Yoga), meditation, mind-body therapy, relaxation, and tai chi.

Medical conditions, such as eczema and asthma are difficult to treat, and sometimes complementary medicine can help when conventional medicine has not been effective.

Homeopathy is accepted as a useful therapy by many doctors, although it should not be used for life-threatening conditions that might require surgery or drugs. The principle of homeopathy is that if a mild dose of a substance is administered, which at full strength would cause symptoms of the illness being treated, the body's defenses, that is, the immune system, will be stimulated to combat the disorder (see Immune System).

Other therapies

Sex therapy is useful when sexual problems are due to a psychological rather than physical reason. The therapy usually involves talking with a therapist, who may suggest exercises for a couple to do at home.

Speech therapy can help people who have speech and communication difficulties; children who have problems are sometimes given play therapy to help them.

See also: **Behavior therapy; Counseling; Gestalt therapy; Group therapy; Meditation; Psychotherapy**

Thermal imaging

Thermal imaging was a diagnostic procedure that was said to record variations in surface temperature. It has proved to be too imprecise, with too many misleading results, and has now been largely abandoned.

When thermal imaging cameras are used to look for survivors after disasters, are they using the same technique as was used when my mother had thermography to diagnose her varicose veins?

Yes. Thermal imaging locates survivors because their body temperature is higher than the temperature of their surroundings and produces images of different intensity. In medicine, thermal imaging, or thermography, used infrared rays emitted by the body to show areas of increased or decreased heat emission, which can indicate tumors, abnormal blood supply, or inflammation.

My sister once had a breast thermogram, and then a mammogram. Why did she have to have two tests?

A breast thermogram was a safe, noninvasive technique that was used to detect abnormalities in the breast. It purported to show tumors as hot spots and cysts as cold spots, but it could not distinguish between benign and malignant tumors, so a patient had to have a mammogram to provide a more accurate diagnosis. Mammography carries a very slight risk of cancer because it uses X rays, so some doctors preferred thermography if they thought the problem was a cyst rather than a tumor.

My father had rheumatoid arthritis and his condition was monitored using thermography. Was this dangerous?

No. Thermography was safe, noninvasive, and nontraumatic. It detected infrared radiation that was naturally emitted. Your father would not be exposed to rays as he would have been with an X ray or a CT scan. Thermography seemed an ideal technique when repeated testing was needed.

Thermal imaging, or thermography, was a diagnostic tool that provided clues to the presence of diseases and abnormalities that altered the temperature of the skin, such as circulatory problems, inflammation, and tumors (see Temperature).

Doctors have used the temperature of the body as an indicator of health for over a hundred years. The internal temperature of a resting healthy person is 98.6°F (37°C), and the body regulates this over a range of environmental temperatures—even though someone may feel cold in winter and hot in summer, his or her internal temperature will stay around 98.6°F.

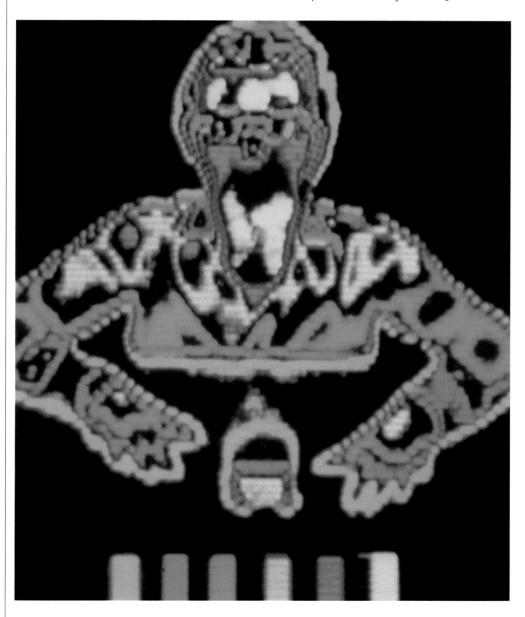

▲ *A thermogram was a color-coded thermal map of skin surface temperature.*

The skin plays a very important part in the regulation process, and its temperature can vary from about 86°F (30°C) to 95°F (35°C) depending on the environmental temperature. Skin temperature is also affected by the movement of air, since air carries heat away from the skin. Internal factors have an effect on skin temperature, because heat is conducted to the surface of the body from structures beneath the skin. These factors formed the basis of thermography.

How did thermography work?

Thermography was a noninvasive technique that attempted to measure temperature distribution over large areas of the surface of the body very quickly without bringing anything into contact with the skin. Every object emits infrared radiation and the intensity of this radiation is related to the temperature of the object—in this case the temperature of the skin surface.

Like visible rays, infrared rays travel in straight lines, and they can be reflected and refracted using mirrors and lenses in the same way as optical devices reflect and refract light. If the infrared rays could be detected and accurately measured, the theory was that the temperature of the object emitting them could be determined. In thermal imaging machines, the infrared radiation was detected by a photosensitive detector. The radiation emanating from a small area of the skin surface was focused into the detector. To allow the machine to view large areas of the skin it was placed up to 10 feet (3 m) away from the patient and oscillating mirrors or rotating prisms were used to scan the whole of the field of view. Temperature distribution was obtained by amplifying a signal from the detector and displaying the result as a varying light level on an oscilloscope or a TV monitor. This picture was then photographed using Polaroid film; the resulting photographs were called thermograms.

What was thermography used for?

The first medical application of thermography was in the 1950s, when it was used by a breast surgeon in the diagnosis of breast disorders. Then its use was expanded into several other areas.

Breast thermography: The influence on the skin temperature of the structures an inch or two below the surface provides information that is useful in the diagnosis of breast disorders. The vessels just below the skin affect the skin temperature and in normal breasts they show up as branching lines on the thermogram because of their higher temperature. The armpits (axillae) also show up as hot regions and in most patients the nipples are shown as cool. In breast cancer the affected area shows up as a hot spot because of an increase in the blood supply to the area and also because of the increased activity of the tumor tissue. A hot spot was not used as a positive diagnosis on its own, it would be substantiated by a mammogram (see Mammography), because in benign breast disease, enlarged blood vessels may also produce hot regions. Cysts will usually show up as well-defined cold regions.

Circulatory problems: Thermography was used in an attempt to assess the efficiency of the blood supply in patients with peripheral vascular disease. Blocked arteries in the lower limbs produce an abnormal skin temperature distribution, which it was hoped would be seen on the thermogram. An attempt to detect varicose veins by this method was also made (see Varicose Veins). The circulation in the brain was monitored by thermography on the premise that changes in the blood supply to the internal and external carotid arteries (that supply the brain) would be reflected in changes in the

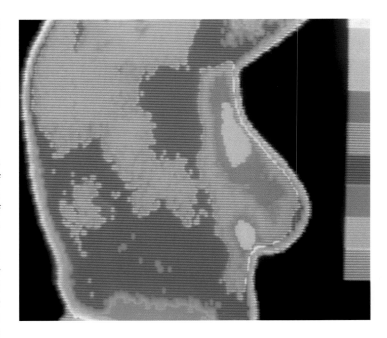

▲ *A thermogram shows the breast. The hottest areas are white, and yellow to red; the coolest are blue, and purple to black.*

temperature of the skin of the face and forehead. Narrowing (stenosis) of the internal carotid artery would show up as cool areas over the eye region and the middle forehead.

Bone and joint disorders: Disorders such as inflammation and bone cancer showed up on thermograms. Thermography showed the rise in temperature in joints affected by rheumatoid arthritis and was useful for monitoring the progress of the disease. Inflammation produced by a slipped disk sometimes showed up, but the results were usually not accurate enough to be useful in diagnosis (see Cancer; Rheumatoid Arthritis; Slipped Disk).

Thyroid disorders: Active thyroid tissue showed as a warm area on a thermogram. Thermography was used to distinguish benign thyroid nodules (adenomas), which show as cold spots, from malignant nodules (thyroid cancer), which show as hot spots. A scan of the thyroid by radioisotopes detects nodules, but cannot distinguish between benign and malignant nodules (see Thyroid).

Results and outlook

Because so many factors affect skin temperature, in most cases the results of thermography were not sufficiently reliable to allow a conclusive diagnosis; further confirmatory tests were needed. For example, in breast disease, thermography was usually carried out with mammography, which is more accurate. However, since mammography uses X rays, there is a slight risk of inducing cancer, especially if the accumulated dose of radiation increases with each examination. Thermography was used regularly without risk to the patient, who was referred for mammography only if the thermogram was doubtful (see X Rays). It was hoped that with further refinement of the equipment it would be possible to obtain sufficiently focused results to make positive and reliable diagnoses. However, this was not so, and thermal imaging for medical purposes has now been virtually abandoned.

See also: Diagnostic imaging

Thirst

Questions and Answers

When it is very hot and I am thirsty, I get much more relief from having a cold drink than a tepid one. Is there a physical reason for this, or is it just psychological?

The amount of fluid your body receives is the same whatever the temperature of the drink you take. However, the relief of thirst depends to a large extent on the stimulation of your mouth and throat as you drink. Cold fluids tend to stimulate the linings here more than tepid fluids. Similarly, hot tea is thirst-quenching even on hot days, again because hotter drinks stimulate the throat more than tepid ones.

My husband has very bad bronchitis and has to breathe through his mouth most of the time. He says this makes him very thirsty. Why does this happen?

One of the things that make us thirsty is that the lining of the throat and mouth gets dry. People with bronchitis or asthmatic attacks who have to breathe through the mouth get very dry in the mouth through evaporation of the water on the lining. This stimulates the thirst centers in the brain, despite the fact that the actual water content of the blood is adequate.

Why do people who have diabetes get so thirsty before the disease is diagnosed and treatment begins?

In diabetics, the main change that occurs in the blood is that there is too much sugar. The problem spills over into the urine, and its presence there prevents the tubules of the kidney from controlling the amount of water that is lost. The most noticeable early indication of diabetes is excessive urine secretion (polyuria), causing the blood to become short of water and resulting in great thirst and an abnormally high fluid intake.

Taking a drink to quench the thirst is not only immensely pleasurable, it is also absolutely vital for people in order for them to maintain adequate amounts of water in the body fluids.

The delicate chemical processes that keep people alive demand that the amount of water in the body is kept very constant. The sense of thirst is one of the most vital human appetites because it ensures that the chemical equilibrium is maintained. Sensitive centers within the brain monitor the amount of water in the blood. These respond quickly to any significant change, producing the sensation of thirst that drives people to seek replenishment when they become short of water.

Remarkably, sensors in the throat seem to be able to assess accurately when a person has drunk enough, even before the centers in the brain signal that the amount of water in the body is adequate. As a symptom, excessive thirst is an important indicator that fluids have been lost. It can point to abnormalities in the kidneys, to the presence of excess sugar in the blood (which causes excess water loss; see Sugars), and to damage to those brain structures that participate in keeping the water balance in order.

The mechanics of thirst

The main control center for the sense of thirst is deep in the brain just below the thalamus and is known as the hypothalamus. Small groups of nerve cells in this gland are sensitive to the amount of water in the blood. If the amount of water in the blood compared with the amount of salts and other substances diminishes, these cells are stimulated and, in addition to producing the hormones that make the kidneys conserve water, produce the sensation of thirst (see Hormones; Salt). These cells are also stimulated by sudden changes in the volume of blood in the circulation, such as occur after a hemorrhage.

The other change that makes people thirsty is that the lining of the mouth and throat becomes dry. This stimulates nerve endings in the lining, which are also connected indirectly with the thirst centers in the hypothalamus. Simply moistening the mouth has a powerful effect in reducing the signals to the brain that fluid is in short supply.

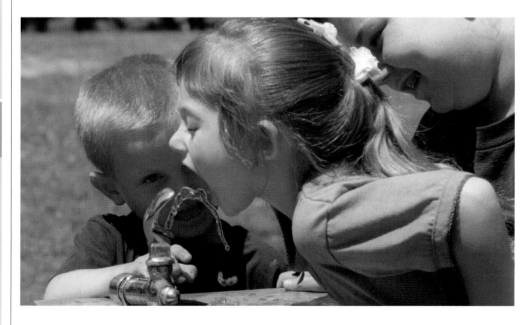

▲ *Water fountains are a convenient way to satiate thirst when other forms of water may not be easily available. While people can remain for long periods without food, regular intake of liquids is vital. Thirst is a sign that a drink is absolutely essential.*

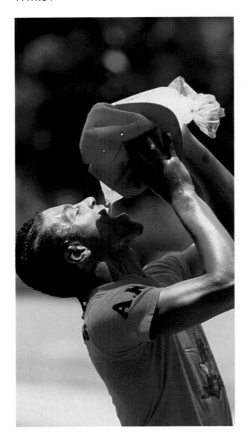

▲ *In hot climates, like those of the southern states, strenuous exercise can cause severe dehydration, so plenty of liquids must be drunk.*

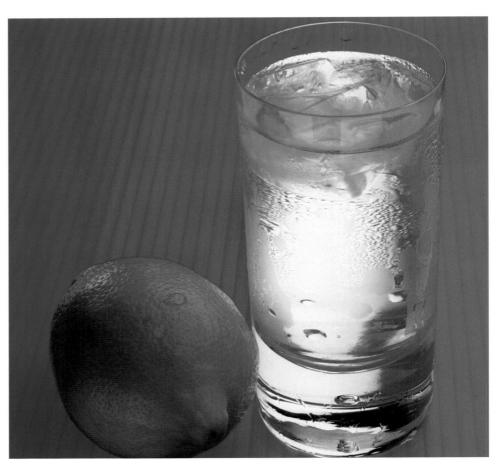

▲ *To some extent, thirst can be stimulated by psychological factors; often the mere sight of a refreshing drink makes us thirsty.*

When people have been deprived of water and are then allowed to drink, they rapidly take enough water to replenish their stock; they stop before the water has had time to be absorbed and change the blood enough to reduce the stimulus to the water-sensitive cells in the hypothalamus. This illustrates the fact that there is some sort of metering mechanism in the body that assesses accurately when a person has drunk enough liquid.

The sensors that control this metering are in the mouth and throat. They coordinate with the thirst center in the brain through relays in the brain stem. In humans, this metering mechanism is not as accurate as it is in other animals, probably because people have superimposed on it certain psychological and habitual factors that are partly in control of our drinking behavior.

Thirst and illness

People are sometimes unable to compensate for dehydration by taking a drink—for example, when they are unconscious and cannot respond to messages from the thirst center in the brain. Thus, when people are very sick they may get dehydrated, especially if they lose fluid by vomiting and diarrhea (see Diarrhea; Vomiting).

Very occasionally, the thirst area in the brain is damaged by a stroke or tumor, and does not respond normally to the changes in the water content of the blood. More often, psychiatric disease, such as certain psychoses, disrupts a person's behavior so much that he or she ignores the signals from the hypothalamus and becomes dehydrated (see

Psychoses). Thirst can be a symptom of various types of disease, and its presence in someone who is sick is often a useful clue to the doctor.

The common factor in people who suffer from abnormal thirst is that they are dehydrated. Dehydration may be brought about because of kidney damage, which may affect the kidney's ability to respond to signals from the brain to retain water. When there is an excess of sugar in the blood, as in diabetes mellitus, the excess spills over into the urine, taking with it an excessive volume of water (see Urinary Tract and Disorders). This is necessary to dissolve and dispose of the abnormally high levels of sugar in the blood. The result is that the blood becomes short of water and this causes great thirst and an abnormally high fluid intake. Once the blood sugar level is controlled by treatment the abnormal thirst will disappear.

In an uncommon disease called diabetes insipidus, the hormone normally produced by the pituitary gland to retain water is inadequately produced or, more rarely, the kidneys themselves may be unable to conserve water.

Internal hemorrhage also produces thirst. This is not so much an aid in diagnosis of the problem as a guide to the treatment (by blood transfusions, for example), since continuing thirst tells the doctors that the effects of the hemorrhage have not been reversed.

See also: **Brain; Diabetes; Hemorrhage; Hypothalamus; Kidneys and kidney diseases; Mouth; Pituitary gland; Throat**

Throat

The air we breathe, as well as food on its way to the digestive tract, has to pass through the throat on its way to the lungs. Any obstruction to this vital passage can represent a serious threat to life.

The lay term "throat" describes the part of the neck between the chin and the collarbones and is the area that leads into the respiratory and digestive tracts. It extends from the oral and nasal cavities to the esophagus and the trachea, and is made up of two main parts: the pharynx and the larynx (see Larynx and Laryngitis; Pharynx).

Structures of the throat

The pharynx is a muscular tube lined with mucous membrane. For practical purposes it is divided into three areas. The part behind the nasal cavity is the nasopharynx, the area behind the mouth the oropharynx, and the area behind the larynx the laryngopharynx. Clumps of lymphoid tissue

ANATOMY OF THE THROAT

The main component of the throat is the pharynx, a muscular tube about 5 in. (13 cm) long stretching from the base of the skull into the esophagus. It is the passage through which everything we eat, drink, and breathe has to pass, the junction point of all nasal and oral passages. It is also connected to the ears by drainage channels—the eustachian tubes—which help to equalize air pressure on each side of the eardrums.

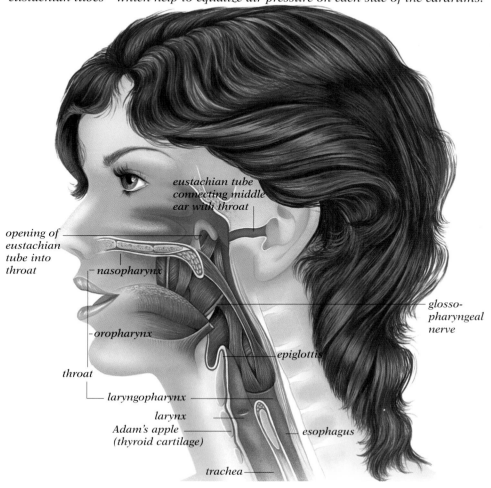

eustachian tube connecting middle ear with throat

opening of eustachian tube into throat

nasopharynx

glosso-pharyngeal nerve

oropharynx

epiglottis

throat

laryngopharynx

larynx

Adam's apple (thyroid cartilage)

esophagus

trachea

Questions and Answers

My husband has been told that he has cancer of the larynx. What are his chances of being cured?

Most forms of cancer of the larynx respond well to treatment. With modern radiotherapy techniques a cure rate of about 90 percent is common. However, the doctors will want to keep a close eye on your husband for the rest of his life, to treat any recurrent problems as they arise.

What is the correct action to take when someone is choking on a bone or a peanut?

Take hold of the person from behind and use a fist to deliver an upward thrust to the abdomen. If the patient is a young child, place him or her face down on the lap and gently thump the child's middle back. Call for help at once.

Why are disorders of the throat often accompanied by pain in one or both ears?

Throat infections may cause pain in the ear because of the phenomenon of pain referral. This occurs when the same nerve supplies the two different but close-lying structures. The patient is unable to discern from which site the pain arises.

My son is always getting ear infections and we have been told that he should have an adenoidectomy. Will this definitely cure him?

It is never possible for a doctor to guarantee that any treatment will be totally successful. However, very enlarged adenoids are frequently implicated in recurrent otitis media (an infection in the middle ear) and it is only right to remove them in the hope that this is the cause of the problem. It is very important to try to minimize infectious attacks in the ear and prevent the deafness that can be associated with them, so if your ear surgeon recommends an adenoidectomy you should seriously consider it.

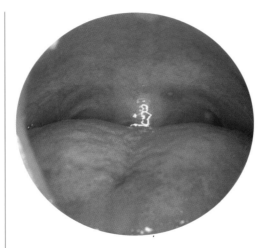

▲ *Caused by the streptococcus bacterium, strep throat is a common throat infection that can be very painful.*

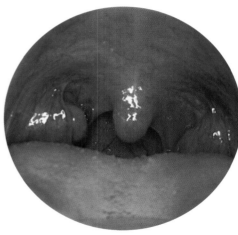

▲ *Infection can spread rapidly in the throat; in this case tonsillitis, usually caused by a streptococcus, has developed.*

lie in the lining of the pharynx; these are the adenoids in the nasopharynx and the tonsils in the oropharynx. They protect the entrance to the food and air passages. The other major part of the throat, the larynx, is in front of the laryngopharynx and is made up of a framework of cartilage swathed in muscles both internally and externally, and lined by a respiratory membrane.

The larynx is a specialized section of the windpipe. It has a flap valve—the epiglottis—hovering over the inlet to the airway, which acts as a type of umbrella against a shower of food and liquid when we eat or drink. The vocal cords are located in the larynx, and held in place by special cartilages. They are suspended across the airway and produce sound when vibrated by air movement (see Vocal Cords).

Functions of the throat

Because the throat is an assembly of different components, it has a variety of functions. First is the pharynx: the channel through which food and liquid enter the digestive tract, and air enters the lungs. The movements of the pharynx must be coordinated to ensure that the respiratory gases end up in the lungs and food and liquid end up in the esophagus. This is achieved by a plexus, or network, of nerves called the pharyngeal plexus, the activity of which is controlled in the lower brain stem, where information is coordinated from the respiratory and swallowing centers higher in the brain (see Brain).

When food is thrown into the oropharynx by the tongue, it is swiftly sent into the esophagus by a wave of muscular contractions that travel down the pharynx (see Esophagus). At the same time mechanisms are triggered to prevent the food from entering the larynx.

No less important are the functions of the larynx, which are to produce sound and to protect the airway. Like the pharynx, the larynx achieves these functions through a complex coordinated nerve supply to its muscles. The nerves that supply the larynx are under the same central influence in the brain as the nerves that supply the pharynx.

Throat disorders

The pharynx and larynx are prone to a number of infections caused by viruses or bacteria, and also to damage by physical agents, such as excessive smoking or drinking. Either of these factors can lead to, for example, chronic laryngitis or pharyngitis. Other throat infections include nasopharyngitis, a viral infection of the mucous membranes lining the nasopharynx. This begins with a burning feeling in the throat that builds up in intensity and is aggravated by speaking and swallowing. The discomfort is accompanied by a general feeling of malaise, which lasts from one to two days. Nasopharyngitis is often confused with tonsillitis. Because the tonsils and the nasopharynx are adjacent to each other, an infection in either area gives rise to similar symptoms. However, in tonsillitis the symptoms are much more severe.

The nasopharynx is also the site of the adenoids, and repeated infections in this area can cause the adenoids to enlarge. Patients with excessively large adenoids are unable to breathe

Home help for a sore throat

A sore throat that accompanies a common cold or other minor infection can be treated at home. Here are some proven remedies that can be tried.

Make up a gargling solution by dissolving two teaspoonfuls of household salt in a cupful of hot, but not boiling, water. Stir until the salt has dissolved, then use the solution to gargle. Make sure you spit the solution out of your mouth when you have finished.

Alternatively, you can use an aspirin gargle by dissolving two soluble aspirin tablets in a cup of hot water. If you swallow this after gargling, the aspirin will relieve some of the pain and reduce any fever you might have.

Drink plenty of hot liquids and try to eat only soft or liquid foods, such as soups, so that you do not take anything into your throat that might cause further damage or inflammation.

Lozenges can be effective in soothing a sore throat and can prevent the throat from becoming dry. Keep the lozenge as far back on your tongue as you can for maximum benefit.

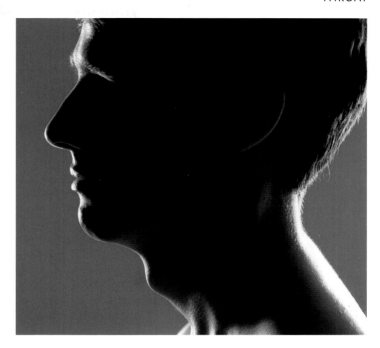

▲ *The thyroid cartilage surrounding the larynx creates the projection called the Adam's apple. It is more prominent in men because they have larger vocal cords.*

through the nose and have a persistently gaping mouth. An increase in adenoid tissue may block the natural drainage channel, the eustachian tube, from the middle ear and cause an accumulation of fluid in this cavity. In severe cases deafness may result, and the condition also predisposes a person to recurrent attacks of otitis media. Children are most affected, and are frequently admitted to the hospital for drainage of the middle ear fluid and removal of the adenoids (see Adenoids).

Papillomatosis is caused by a virus that affects the larynx; it occurs in children and adults. The virus is similar to that which produces warts on the skin. As the papillomas increase in size they restrict the passage of air and may even choke the patient. Like warts on the skin, the growths can disappear spontaneously, but in severe cases surgery is required to remove them.

Pharyngeal cancer

Cancer of the pharynx is an unusual condition that occurs in middle and old age. Patients complain of a progressively painful difficulty in swallowing. The pain is experienced not only at the site of the disease but also radiating to the ear. In a large number of patients a lump appears on one side of the neck. Although cancer of the pharynx is an extremely serious condition, a high proportion of patients can be greatly helped by either radiotherapy or surgery (see Radiotherapy; Surgery).

Laryngeal cancer

Cancer of the larynx is a more common throat cancer. It is a form of cancer that can be cured if the disease is diagnosed and treated early. It occurs most frequently in late middle age and is much more common in men than in women. Most patients are, or have been, heavy smokers for much of their life (see Cancer). Progressive hoarseness is the most common symptom, and patients may also complain of an odd feeling in the throat, slight difficulty in breathing, pain in their ear, or pain radiating from the throat to the ear. Occasionally they may cough up a small amount of blood.

Most cases can be cured by a course of radiotherapy. However, in a few cases the disease recurs or fails to respond to radiation treatment and surgery is necessary.

Foreign objects in the throat

A wide variety of foreign objects have been found in the pharynx, ranging from fish bones to coins and bottle tops. Any foreign object in the throat is potentially dangerous because it can perforate the pharyngeal wall and set up serious infection in the surrounding tissues of the throat.

Patients who have swallowed a foreign object that has become lodged in the throat are rarely in any doubt about its presence; every attempt to swallow even their own saliva is excruciatingly painful. If the object is lodged high in the pharynx it can usually be removed in the emergency room of a hospital. However, if it is lodged lower down—for example, in the laryngopharynx—it must be removed under general anesthesia.

Foreign bodies that are inhaled into the larynx can threaten a patient's life and little time should be lost in getting treatment. The younger the patient the more serious the condition, since the diameter of a child's airway is so narrow that even a small object is likely to obstruct it totally.

Removal of any object from the larynx is a matter of surgical urgency, and may require a temporary tracheostomy (an artificial opening in the trachea) to protect the lower airway and maintain adequate breathing. Recovery from this surgery is swift (see Tracheostomy).

See also: Neck; Otitis; Sore throat; Tonsils

Thrombosis

Questions and Answers

Will quitting smoking really help to lessen my chance of suffering from a coronary thrombosis?

If you smoke cigarettes, you stand a far greater chance of having a heart attack as well as developing chronic bronchitis or cancer. As soon as a person quits smoking, the chance of contracting these life-threatening conditions is believed to decrease. Five years after stopping smoking, a reformed smoker is at no greater risk from a heart attack than someone who has never smoked.

Is it true that some doctors prescribe rat poison as a treatment for thrombosis?

The anticoagulant drug warfarin is also used to kill rats and mice. This group of anticoagulants was discovered when cattle feeding on sweet clover were found to be suffering from bruising and hemorrhages. A powerful anticoagulant was discovered in the plants on which the cattle were grazing. Warfarin is prescribed in very small doses commonly to prevent thrombosis. Clotting is monitored by a doctor, who usually orders a blood test every few weeks.

I am thinking of going on the Pill. Can it cause thrombosis?

There tends to be a higher incidence of thrombosis in women who take a high-dosage oral contraceptive, particularly if they are over 35, are overweight, and smoke. However, the modern low-dosage estrogen Pill has only a very small risk of causing thrombosis—indeed a smaller chance than in pregnancy itself. Of those who develop thrombotic side effects, the majority suffer from thrombophlebitis of the legs, and should immediately see a doctor and arrange to start some alternative form of birth control.

Heart attacks, strokes, and even varicose veins all have a single cause—a thrombosis, which is a blood clot in an artery or a vein that blocks circulation. Can anything be done to minimize the risk of thrombosis?

People who smoke, those who are obese, and diabetics are more prone to thrombotic diseases, but these diseases can occur among the healthy. However, risks can be reduced and preventative measures can be taken.

Thrombus formation

The blood forms a clot (or thrombus) as a normal, healthy protective process by which bleeding from a damaged blood vessel is stopped and the repair process begins. There are three stages in the process of stopping bleeding from a small blood vessel; constriction, formation of a platelet plug, and clotting. As soon as bleeding begins, the damaged vessel constricts, slowing blood flow and attracting platelets to the site of the damage. Platelets are tiny cell fragments that become sticky and adhere to each other and to the lining of the vessel, temporarily plugging the hole. Finally, a clot will form. Thromboplastin, an extract from the blood vessel wall, oozes from the torn edges of the vessel. This starts a chain reaction in which fibrinogen, a soluble blood protein, is changed into long strands of fibrin, forming a meshwork to trap passing red blood cells and platelets. In the last stage of clot formation, the fibrin mesh tightens, fluid is squeezed out of the clot, and the torn vessel walls pull together (see Blood).

How a thrombosis occurs

When blood circulation through the heart, limbs, or brain is sluggish, or the blood contains an excess of clotting factors, or the blood vessels are affected by atheroma, a clot may block a major artery or vein. The thrombosis may occur in different parts of the body.

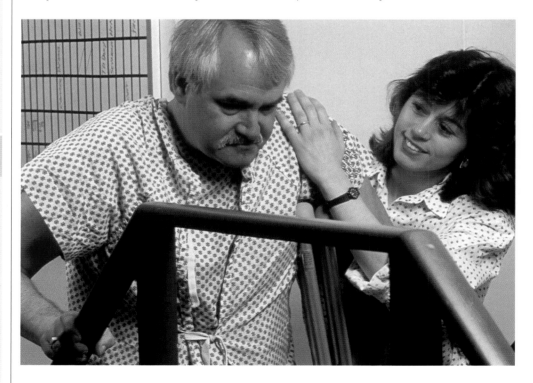

▲ *Doctors encourage patients to become mobile as soon as possible after surgery, to reduce the likelihood of vein thrombosis.*

When thrombosis occurs in one of the coronary arteries of the heart, a patient will have a heart attack or myocardial infarction. Thrombosis in the brain results in a stroke. If thrombosis develops in a leg vein it causes phlebitis, and if it occurs in an artery supplying a limb it may result in gangrene (see Gangrene).

An embolism occurs when a thrombus forming in a major blood vessel, or on the lining of the heart, breaks loose. It is swept away by the bloodstream and becomes lodged in a narrow vessel, completely cutting off the blood supply to part of the lung or brain, or to an arm or leg. Because of the anatomy of the circulatory system, thrombosis in a leg vein may break loose to form a pulmonary embolism in the lung. If the clot originates from a neck artery, it may be carried into the brain to produce a cerebral embolism (see Circulatory System).

Why does a thrombosis occur?

Thrombosis nearly always results from one or a combination of the following: cardiovascular disease, prolonged immobilization, the aftermath of major surgery, pregnancy, or the Pill.

Some individuals are more susceptible to thrombosis than others. In these cases there is usually both an abnormality of blood vessels and a hypercoagulable state in which the blood has a tendency to clot more easily than normal. Any attempt to reduce the risk of thrombosis must entail either preventing or correcting the disease in the heart or blood vessels, or reducing the ease with which clotting occurs in the blood.

Disorders of the blood vessels

As people grow older, signs of degenerative disease become more marked in the major arteries. Pathologists describe this degenerative process as atheroma, and the effect on the blood

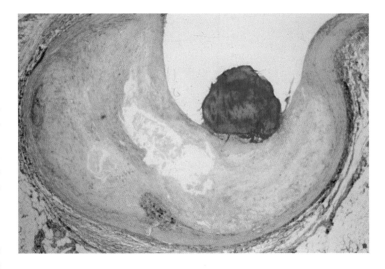

▲ *One of the most common places for a clot to form is in the heart. This cross section of a coronary artery clearly shows a small clot that has grown within it.*

vessels as atherosclerosis, or hardening of the arteries. Atherosclerosis is most likely to occur first in the heart and the major arteries, where the arteries are subjected to the most stress. Not surprisingly, if blood pressure is abnormally high, then atherosclerosis develops early in the blood vessels supplying the heart, brain, and limbs. The arteries become narrower and more rigid, significantly reducing the flow of blood.

Atheroma in its earliest form can be detected in childhood. Tiny yellowish flecks develop in the linings of the major arteries, particularly where they branch or split into smaller tributaries. By middle age the flecks have become distinct streaks that are rich in cholesterol. The lining of the vessel may then become roughened and cracked. Platelets are attracted to the cracked surface and a small clot may grow into the cavity of the artery. This may create a turbulence in blood flow, which may finally tear the clot loose, resulting in a dangerous embolism of the brain or the limbs.

The chambers of the heart are a common place for clots to form, particularly in the heart valves. This is especially likely to happen if the valves are already damaged or narrowed. Rheumatic fever in childhood is still the most common cause of valvular disease, although this condition is rare in today's children.

Some people in the middle or older age group are suffering from illness brought on by an attack of rheumatic fever in childhood (see Rheumatic Fever).

A thrombus may form in the heart's atria if they are beating irregularly or fibrillating. Occasionally, after a severe coronary thrombosis, a whole area of the left ventricle, the main pumping chamber of the heart, becomes thin and wasted, and fails to

▼ *No matter what age you are, quitting smoking, keeping to a healthy balanced diet, and getting regular exercise will help to reduce the risk of thrombosis.*

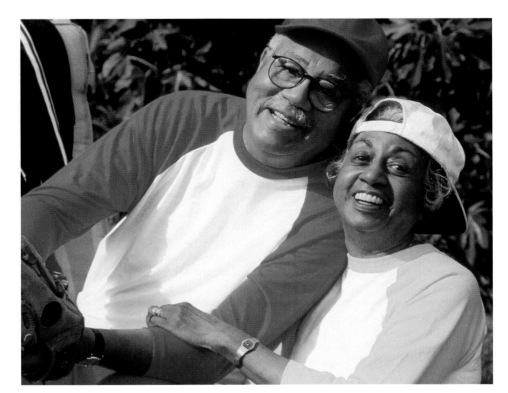

A friend told me that you can get gangrene from a blood clot. Is she correct?

Indirectly, yes. Gangrene occurs when living muscle and skin are deprived of blood supply and die. Dry gangrene often occurs when a blood clot blocks the blood flow in an artery supplying blood to an arm or a leg. Fingers or toes are usually affected first by discoloration, cold, and sometimes pain. Eventually, the digits may turn black and the gangrene spreads up the limb to a level that is determined by the site of the blockage.

I had rheumatic fever as a child and have been told by my doctor that I have a damaged heart valve. He has prescribed an anticoagulant drug for me. Why is this necessary?

Rheumatic fever was once a very common childhood disease. It is less common now, but many sufferers have been left with narrowed or stiffened heart valves. These produce murmurs, or abnormal sounds, which are detected during a medical examination. Damaged valves often interfere with the pumping action of the heart and can lead to irregularities of heart rhythm. Both these complications can result in blood clotting in the chambers of the heart. To make the blood clot more slowly, and prevent clots from forming, anticoagulant drugs such as warfarin are prescribed. Often the only way to improve the action of the heart and prevent further damage is to replace the faulty valve with a metal or plastic valve. Replacement valves still need anticoagulant protection, and patients usually remain on warfarin or similar drugs.

How did the word "thrombosis" come about?

It is derived from the ancient Greek language and means a "curdling" or a "coagulation." Its first known use in English was around 1706.

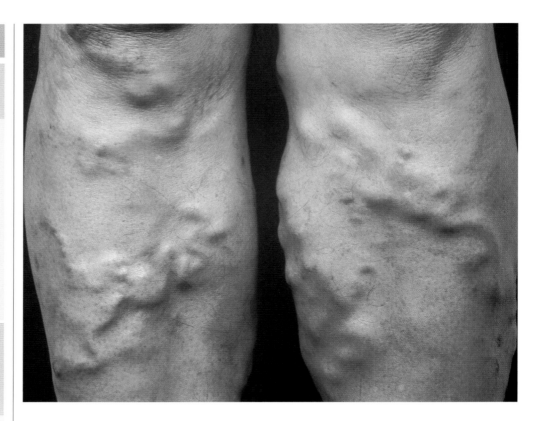

▲ *One of the most common causes of thrombosis is varicose veins, which are a problem for some pregnant women. The veins can often cause itching, sometimes pain, and, although rarely, skin ulceration. The symptoms can be alleviated by taking frequent rests and by wearing support hose.*

To prevent thrombotic diseases
Quit smoking.
If you are overweight, start to rid yourself of those extra pounds.
Diabetics should stick religiously to their diet and take their medication.
Attend a prenatal clinic regularly for checkups if you are pregnant.
After an operation, follow your doctor's orders and get active as soon as possible.
Don't cut down on your medication if you feel well but suffer from high blood pressure.
Embark on a program of regular exercise; a thrombosis is much less common in individuals who are fit and active, regardless of age.

contract effectively. This is a likely site for a thrombus which all too often leads to a serious embolism (see Heart).

Coronary thrombosis

Coronary thrombosis is a common cause of what is generally called a heart attack; doctors usually refer to a heart attack as myocardial infarction.

One person in three will be affected by coronary artery disease, and heart disease was the leading cause of death in 2002 in the United States. Until the age of 70, about four times as many men as women suffer a coronary thrombosis. Women over 70 are just as likely to be affected as men (see Heart Attack; Heart Disease).

Those most at risk of a heart attack are male, are overweight, eat a diet that is rich in saturated fats, and lead a stressful life with minimal exercise.

In addition, diabetics, and people whose families have a history of heart attacks, are also prone to heart disease. However, the biggest group of risk takers is smokers; a cigarette smoker is five times more likely to suffer a heart attack than a nonsmoker.

Thrombotic diseases

DISEASE	CAUSES	SYMPTOMS	DANGERS	TREATMENT	PREVENTION
Coronary thrombosis	Stress. High blood pressure. Diabetes. Atherosclerosis.	Faintness. Breathlessness. Increasing, crushing chest pain.	Irregular heartbeat. Low blood pressure. Congestion of the lungs. Other thromboses.	Aspirin. Bed rest. Pain relief. Oxygen. Drugs to stabilize heart rhythm and blood pressure.	Quit smoking. Lose weight. Get regular exercise. Avoid stress.
Cerebral thrombosis and embolism	Heart disease. High blood pressure. Also atherosclerosis.	One-sided weakness of the face, arm and leg, or both. Loss of feeling. Drowsiness. Difficulty with speech. Unsteadiness.	Chest infection. Pressure sores. Stiffening of joints. Depression.	Retraining exercises. Speech therapy. Anticoagulant drugs.	Quit smoking. Have your blood pressure checked frequently.
Venous thrombosis	Immobilization. Major surgery. Varicose veins. Pregnancy and occasionally the contraceptive pill.	Pain and swelling. Also tenderness. Discoloration of the lower leg.	Pleurisy. Massive embolism of the lung. Postphlebitic limb.	Rest and elevation of the limb. Support hose. Exercise. Anticoagulant drugs.	Patients with varicose veins: wear support hose. Phlebitis sufferers: seek specialist advice during pregnancy, or before starting the Pill or undergoing surgery.
Arterial thrombosis and embolism	Diabetes. Smoking. Heart disease. Also atherosclerosis.	Limb pain. Numbness and cold. Blackening of fingers or toes.	Gangrene	Bed rest. Surgery. Anticoagulant drugs.	Quit smoking. Diabetes sufferers: stick closely to diet.

Causes, symptoms, and treatment of coronary disease

The two coronary arteries embedded in the muscular walls of the heart divert oxygen-rich blood, fresh from the lungs, to small vessels that feed all parts of the heart muscle. It is vital that these arteries remain open; even a slight narrowing may cause symptoms during times of exertion.

Persons at risk of coronary disease have a tendency to form fatty deposits that roughen the lining of the arteries and narrow the central channel. If a blockage occurs gradually, the person may experience pain only on exertion. This is typical of the pain of angina, and usually it is severe enough to make the sufferer stop what he or she is doing. The angina pain then subsides. Although it is often frightening, it serves as a warning, making the sufferer rest long enough for blood flow to be restored to the oxygen-starved muscle before serious damage can be done, and allowing time for new circulatory channels to open up over the following weeks.

When a coronary thrombosis develops at a site of narrowing, it may completely block the blood supply to part of the heart muscle. That part will be so severely damaged it will cease to contract normally; the symptoms, then, will be sudden and severe. Patients experience crushing chest pain, which is sometimes also felt in the arm and jaw; they may feel breathless and sweat profusely. These symptoms do not always begin when the person is being particularly energetic, and do not usually improve even when he or she is resting.

Coronary thrombosis almost always requires treatment in the hospital, though patients will be allowed out of bed for short periods within the first two weeks and will embark on a program of graduated exercise. It is believed that once a firm scar has replaced the damaged heart muscle, exercise will encourage the formation of new channels to replace the thrombosed artery (see Exercise).

Cerebral thrombosis

Strokes are one of the most common causes of death and disablement. Those most at risk are people who suffer from high blood pressure, are diabetics, have a high serum cholesterol, or smoke. Strokes may run in families. Some people with heart disease are predisposed to strokes (see Stroke).

Causes, symptoms, and treatment of stroke

A stroke can be caused by bleeding from a weakened artery into the brain (cerebral hemorrhage), a sudden blockage of an artery by a flake of material that has come adrift from a diseased artery or from the heart (embolism), or a more gradual blockage of an artery by clot formation within a diseased artery of the brain (cerebral thrombosis). The arterial disease that predisposes people to all three types of stroke is atherosclerosis (see Arteries and Artery Disease).

The effects of a stroke depend entirely on the size and situation of the affected area of the brain. If the right side of the brain is damaged, there is usually weakness, paralysis of the facial muscles,

Questions and Answers

Six months ago I had deep vein thrombosis which was a complication of my hysterectomy. Now my leg still swells from time to time. Is this usual?

The valves in the veins in the legs allow blood to flow against gravity toward the heart, but prevent backflow stagnation of blood in the lower legs and feet. When a blood clot forms in these veins, the valves are often damaged. The clot is eventually digested and removed by enzymes in the blood, and blood flow is restored. For many weeks after the thrombosis, increased pressure may force fluid into the tissues, causing the legs to swell, notably after a person stands for a long time. If you've had deep vein thrombosis, avoid standing for long periods, try to do some walking, and wear support hose. These measures may help to relieve the symptoms.

Can varicose veins be dangerous or are they just unsightly?

Varicose veins are rarely more than an unsightly nuisance. Some people can develop painful, hard, red swollen areas known as superficial thrombophlebitis. Varicose veins increase the danger of a deep vein thrombosis after surgery or pregnancy. It is not uncommon for a cut or fall to cause serious bleeding from a prominent varicose vein. If you suffer from varicose veins, avoid prolonged standing and wear special support hose. In serious cases, surgery may be required to deal with the condition.

A woman at work suffers from phlebitis. What is it?

Phlebitis is an inflammation of a vein, usually in the leg, resulting in a blood clot in the vein. It is fairly painful, and the area may be red, swollen, and tender to the touch. Phlebitis does usually disappear in a week or two without any serious consequences, but there may be recurrent attacks throughout a person's life.

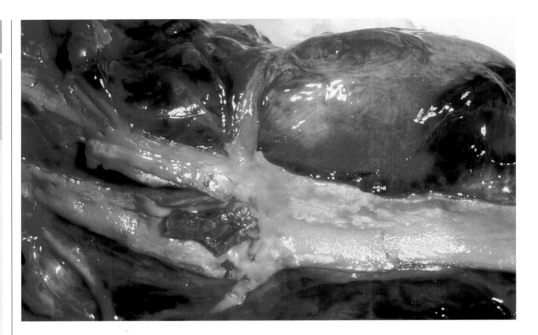

▲ *A thrombosis can sometimes be fatal: here a clot has completely enveloped the internal carotid artery in the neck.*

and loss of sensation in the left arm and leg. If the left side of the brain is affected, the patient may lose total or partial control of speech and be paralyzed on the right side of the body (see Brain Damage and Disease).

Cerebral thrombosis produces sudden paralysis or weakness that begins to improve within hours after the stroke occurs. Recovery is helped by early encouragement of the patient, and physical therapy or speech therapy or both. A high proportion of stroke victims make a full recovery, but in the remainder, the degree of recuperation will depend on the severity of the initial damage to the brain.

Causes, symptoms, and treatment of thrombophlebitis

Phlebitis is an inflammation of a vein; it is usually associated with a blockage of the vein by a blood clot. The clot forms in a limb, most frequently in the leg and, rarely, in the arm.

Thrombophlebitis can affect either a superficial vein or a deep vein. The most common cause of superficial thrombophlebitis is varicose veins. The veins lie directly under the skin and at points connect with the deeper veins. If the blood flow is sluggish, or the vein is traumatized, the veins will become inflamed and clotting may occur. In most cases, varicose veins, which are more common in women than in men, are no more than an unsightly nuisance. They are made worse by standing and by pregnancy, and often cause itching, sometimes pain, and rarely ulceration of the skin.

At times they can cause more serious problems, especially during pregnancy or when a patient is confined to bed by some immobilizing illness or after surgery. The veins may then become painful and hard. The inflammation usually disappears on its own, but a hot water bottle will give relief.

Deep vein thrombosis

Deep vein thrombophlebitis is more serious and is likely to occur in varicose vein sufferers. When varicose veins are so large that most of the blood being pumped back from the legs to the heart is carried in dilated veins beneath the skin, the blood flow through the main leg veins can be so slow that it encourages formation of an extensive clot. The thrombus, in addition to causing a painful, hot, swollen limb, can permanently damage the valves controlling blood flow toward the heart and against the force of gravity. In the majority of patients the thrombosis resolves completely and normal blood circulation is restored, but in a few the aching and swelling of the limb may recur on prolonged standing.

See also: **Inflammation; Physical therapy; Speech therapy; Valves; Varicose veins**

Thrush

"Thrush" is the common term for what is medically known as candidiasis—an infection with a fungus of the genus Candida. It is one of the most common human infections and is usually of minor importance.

Questions and Answers

Isn't thrush just an infection of babies' mouths?

Thrush is common in babies, but it is by no means confined to them, nor to their mouths. It can involve both the exterior and the interior of the body and is as common in the diaper area as in the mouth.

What is a mucous membrane, and what is its connection with thrush?

All the surfaces of the body are covered with a special nonstick layer. The outside layer is the epidermis of the skin. The inside layer is the mucous membrane, of which the most accessible parts are in the mouth, nose, and genital area. Thrush fungus grows well on mucous membranes, so it is commonly found in these areas.

Why do diabetics often get thrush?

Diabetics have sugar in their urine, and the thrush fungus thrives on carbohydrates. In female diabetics, especially, there is a risk of thrush in the area around the urinary outlet and vagina, which, once established, can spread widely.

Why are people with AIDS especially prone to thrush?

The thrush fungus can be found everywhere, but a healthy immune system easily combats such minor infections. If the immune system is not working properly, as in AIDS, many infections can become established, especially thrush.

Is thrush caused by a single kind of fungus?

No, there are many different species, but they are all similar in appearance and effect. Most cases of thrush in otherwise healthy people are caused by two Candida species of fungi.

Thrush infections are far more common in people than is generally supposed. The fungus is present in the mouth, throat, and intestines of 50 percent of people in the United States. It is present in the vagina of 30 percent of pregnant women and 20 percent of nonpregnant women, and on the skin of 5 percent of all people. These figures indicate that thrush is predominantly an infection of the body's internal membranes rather than of the skin (see Membranes).

The Candida genus contains many different species, most of which can affect human beings. The majority of human thrush infections are caused by either *C. albicans* or *C. tropicalis*.

Candida gets its name from the typical white curdy appearance of the fungus when it is present on mucous membranes (see Mucus). The Latin term *candida* is the feminine form of *candidus*, meaning "white." Some of the other Candida species, such as *C. parapsilosis*, *C. guilliermondii*, and *C. krusei*, mainly affect people with immune deficiency problems.

Candida fungus can exist in a yeastlike form that reproduces by budding, or in a form known as a mycelium of a mass of branching filaments (hyphae) that spread throughout any area that provides suitable nutrients. The yeastlike pattern is most common in immunocompromised people and in those receiving treatment with antifungal drugs in whom the underlying factors encouraging thrush have not been dealt with. It is also common in people who have acquired their infection from tubes which were passed into the body for surgical purposes and which were then left in place for long periods of time. The mycelium form, however, is the most persistent and hardest to treat—the fungus adheres tenaciously to human tissues and surgical equipment. The risk of serious thrush infections in people who are in none of these categories is very small.

Thrush infections are common in the hospital because hospital patients often have surgical incisions, and transfusion, drainage, and other tubes that breach the surface of the body. They are also commonly given broad-spectrum antibiotics. Although there are antifungal drugs effective against the common species of Candida, some of the strains that occur in hospital-acquired infections are able to resist these drugs.

Severity

The severity of a thrush infection depends on the amount of nutrient available to the fungus. Candida fungus lives on glucose or glycogen, the storage form of glucose. If these nutrients are

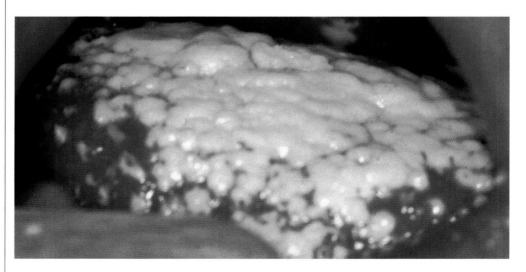

▲ *Thrush is very common in babies, occurring in the mouth (above) or diaper area.*

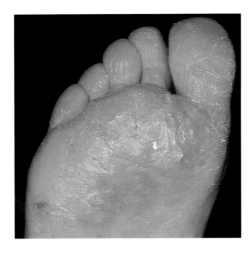

▲ *A thrush infection may occur on the soles of the feet, particularly in people with sweaty feet. It can be successfully treated with an antifungal cream.*

The risk of thrush

The people most likely to acquire thrush are:

People with diabetes

Pregnant women

Women using oral contraceptives

Intravenous drug abusers

People with AIDS

Those with other forms of immune system disorders

Those on immunosuppressive drugs for organ transplants

People on long-term, large-dosage steroid drugs

Those taking long-term antibiotics

People with leukemia

People with cancer

present in the body's secretions the fungus will grow and spread.

Glucose and glycogen are present in higher quantities on the mucous membranes of pregnant women, women taking oral contraceptives, people with diabetes, and people taking steroid drugs. People whose diabetes is well controlled and who keep their urine largely free from glucose are much less likely to develop thrush than those whose diabetes is poorly controlled; if they do contract it, it will be less severe (see Diabetes). Similarly, people on low-dosage steroids are less likely to develop severe thrush than those on long-term, high-dosage steroids.

Broad-spectrum antibiotics can kill most bacteria but they have no effect on fungi. Their effect on the bodily secretions is to prevent the usage of glucose by other organisms and to leave more available for the Candida species present. They may also destroy helpful bacteria, such as the lactobacilli of the vagina, which produce an acid (lactic acid) that is harmful to the thrush fungi and other organisms.

Effects of thrush

On mucous membranes such as the inside of the mouth or in the genital area, thrush appears as separate, raised, white patches on an inflamed base. These may cause pain but are often symptomless. If the fungus spreads down into the esophagus there may be severe pain behind the breastbone, with pain and difficulty in swallowing.

Women with vaginal thrush will usually have a creamy or cheesy vaginal discharge, severe itching, pain on sexual intercourse, and pain on urination (see Itches). Sexual partners are readily infected. Vaginal thrush is most common during pregnancy, and in women who are taking oral contraceptives. A high proportion of cases of mucosal and vaginal thrush occur after a course of antibiotics has been taken.

Thrush of the skin most commonly affects the groin, the armpits, and the skin between the buttocks and under the breasts. The affected areas are moist and red with irregular margins. Many small satellite areas, like little blisters, commonly surround the main patches of infection. The skin around the nails may also become infected, especially if it is allowed to remain constantly wet. Thrush of the nails results in reddened, swollen, and painful nail folds, sometimes with exuding pus. If neglected, the nails themselves may become thickened, hard, yellow, and discolored, and may separate from the nail bed (see Nails).

Chronic mucocutaneous thrush is a form of thrush that affects the skin, the nails, the hair, and the mucous membranes, and it is particularly persistent. About half the people with this form have an underactive thyroid gland (see Thyroid). This is a strange form of immune deficiency that is limited to defense against Candida species and some of the other fungus skin infections. There is no problem with other types of infections, and the condition, although distressing, is limited to the skin, its appendages, and the adjoining mucous membrane surfaces.

It is only in people with severe immune deficiency that thrush may become a life-threatening condition. In such cases the fungus can affect any organ or part of the body. For example, it is common for the Candida fungus to settle inside one or both eyes, where it can severely damage vision. Fungus infection of the inside of the heart is also common in immune deficiency. These widespread infections are most likely to occur in immunocompromised people who have to be artificially tube-fed or who require long-term fluid infusions into the bloodstream.

Treatment

The first step in successful treatment of thrush is to remove, if possible, the underlying factor or factors that are encouraging the infection. There is little point, for instance, in repeatedly applying antifungal creams in a case of genital thrush in an uncontrolled diabetic. For the great majority of cases of minor thrush, however, local treatment with such creams will be highly effective.

Mucous membrane or skin thrush will respond readily to creams or lotions containing antifungal drugs such as clotrimazole, nystatin, or miconazole. For more serious internal infections and for very severe external infections, treatment by mouth is often necessary. A single dose of the drug fluconazole is capable of curing most cases of vaginal thrush. However, it is sometimes necessary for the woman's sexual partner to be treated also. Persistent infections of the mouth may require the use of lozenges of clotrimazole. Gargling with suspensions of antifungal drugs is also useful. Suitable pediatric medication is available for babies and children.

In all cases the treatment of thrush is a matter for a doctor and should be undertaken only by a patient who is under medical supervision.

See also: **Diaper rash; Infection and infectious diseases; Mouth; Vagina; Vaginal discharge; Yeast infections**

Thymus

At one time, the role of the thymus in the body was a mystery. However research over the years has shown that it plays a vital role in the body's defenses against disease.

Questions and Answers

Is it possible to live without a thymus?

After the age of puberty, as we begin to grow older, the thymus starts to shrink. It may not be found in elderly people. This is because it has set up lifelong immunity. Normally, in the first few years of life, we will have come into contact with, and gained immunity to, most of the infections that the immune system is designed to repel. If a baby is born with an inadequate or absent thymus, he or she will not be able to fight infection. The thymus is essential early in life, but it can be removed later.

My husband said he had X-ray treatment for his thymus when he was a baby because it was too big. Is this common?

It is no longer the practice to irradiate large thymus glands in children. Before the importance of the thymus gland to immunity was realized, it was a common treatment.

My brother has myasthenia, and the doctors want to remove his thymus. I thought myasthenia was a nervous system disease, and I don't see the relevance of a gland in the chest. Please explain.

Myasthenia is a nervous system disorder and symptoms include weakness and tiredness of the muscles, which get worse during the day. The disease is caused by the formation of antibodies to the junctions between the nerves and muscles by the body's own immune system. These antibodies attack the junction, and the nerves cannot instruct the muscles to move. Since the thymus is very much involved with the control of the immune system, it has been found that removing the thymus can be effective in helping some myasthenia sufferers.

Over the last two decades it has become clear that the thymus sits at the center of a remarkable web of interconnected organs and tissues that make up the immune system, which defends the body from attack by infection.

There are still some questions about exactly how the thymus does its job, but it is now known to be essential for the proper running of the immune system, and its major function is carried out during the first few years of life.

Where is it?

The thymus is found in the upper part of the chest, where it lies just behind the breastbone (sternum). It consists of two lobes that join in front of the windpipe (trachea). In a young adult it measures a few centimeters in length and weighs about ½ ounce (15 g). However, unlike any other organ in the body, it is at its largest at around the time of puberty, when it may weigh as much as 1½ ounces (43 g).

In a baby, the thymus is very large compared with the rest of the body, and it may extend quite a long way down the chest behind the breastbone. It grows quickly until about the age of seven, after which it grows more slowly until the child reaches puberty (see Puberty).

After the age of puberty the thymus starts to shrink in size in a process called involution, until in an elderly person the only thymus tissue present may be merely a small amount of fat and connective tissue.

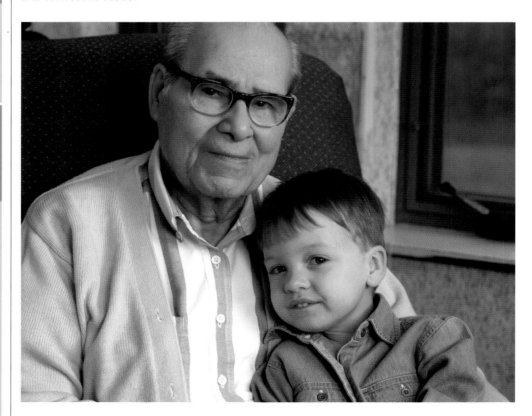

▲ *The thymus is at its most vigorous in the first years of youth, setting up immunity to disease; its function fulfilled, it shrinks into insignificance in old age.*

SIZE AND LOCATION OF THE THYMUS

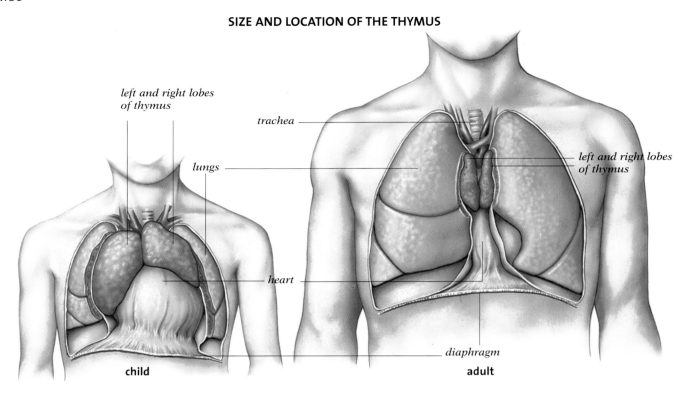

left and right lobes
of thymus

trachea

lungs

left and right lobes
of thymus

heart

diaphragm

child　　　　　**adult**

▲ *The relative sizes of the thymus in an adult and a child demonstrate its importance in establishing the body's immune system early in life. In adulthood it actually shrinks.*

Structure and function

The thymus is made up of lymphoid tissue, epithelium, and fat. The lymphoid tissue consists of many small round cells called lymphocytes, which are the basic unit of the immune system. These cells are also found in the blood, the bone marrow, the lymph glands, and the spleen, and they travel into the tissues as part of the inflammatory reaction.

The outer layer of the thymus, which is called the cortex, has many lymphocytes. Inside this is an area called the medulla, which contains lymphocytes and also other sorts of thymus cells.

In the early years of life, the thymus is concerned with programming the way in which the immune system works. It is now known that the thymus is responsible for many of the most important aspects of the immune system. There are two main sorts of immune cells in the body and both are different types of lymphocytes. The first type are T or thymus cell lymphocytes that are controlled by the thymus and are responsible for the recognition of foreign substances and for many of the ways in which the body attacks them. The second type are B lymphocytes, which are responsible for making antibodies to foreign substances.

The exact ways in which the thymus goes about controlling the T lymphocytes are not known, but it certainly processes the T cells. One important mechanism has come to

light. It seems that about 95 percent of the new types of lymphocyte that are made in the thymus are in fact destroyed there, before they ever have an opportunity to get out into the rest of the body. The probable reason for this is that they would have the potential for turning against the body itself, and the only cells that the thymus allows to develop are those that attack foreign substances.

The T cell processing in early life is affected by the environment to which the baby is exposed. This modulation of the T cells occurs in the thymus and its effect is that babies who are unduly protected against infection and other similar hazards may, later in life, have a less efficient immune system. Babies brought up on a farm, for instance, are less likely to develop asthma later.

As an isolated organ, the thymus rarely causes any trouble. However, it is important to remember that the T lymphocytes it controls are the most central part of the body's immune system, and therefore extremely important in almost all serious diseases.

In the thymus itself, as opposed to the wider aspects of its function, two main problems may occur. First, the thymus may fail to develop properly in babies. As might be expected, this leads to a failure of the immune system and a failure to resist infection, which may prove fatal. This, however, is not a common problem. Second, tumors can occur in the thymus. These are called thymomas, and they are treated by surgery followed by X-ray treatment (see Surgery; Tumors).

▲ *Low-power magnification of a section through a normal thymus shows large purple masses, which are the lobes of this vital organ.*

See also: **Immune system; Lymphocytes**

Thyroid

Questions and Answers

I am very nervous and anxious all the time and irritable with my children. Is it possible that I have an overactive thyroid?

Yes, although it may be difficult to differentiate between symptoms of the disease and those of pure anxiety. An overactive thyroid disorder is associated with weight loss, and the characteristic protruding eyes of Graves' disease, which is the main form of thyrotoxicosis or overactive thyroid. If you find that you are shaky and have a lot of difficulty tolerating heat, then your thyroid may be the reason. The tests for thyrotoxicosis are straightforward and if your doctor suspects this might be the trouble, he or she will arrange for you to have a blood test to confirm the diagnosis.

I have an overactive thyroid and am about to see a specialist. I'm scared of surgery; is there another treatment I could try?

You may be advised to have surgery, although your worries might lead the doctor to suggest alternative treatment. First, you could be given pills to take for about 18 months to suppress the activity of the gland. However, the condition might recur in the future. Second, you could be given treatment with radioiodine (radioactive iodine that is taken up by the thyroid), which reduces the level of thyroid activity. This has the advantage of being simple, and the condition is unlikely to recur. However, this type of treatment is not given to very young people or to women who might become pregnant, since there is a theoretical risk that it will cause cancer in the patient or in any children that may subsequently be born. There is also a definite risk of underactivity of the thyroid after treatment, but this, in turn, is very easy to control.

Problems associated with the thyroid and the hormone it produces are fairly common. However, many of the disorders respond extremely well to treatment and can be completely cured once they have been identified.

Section through thyroid

Problems associated with the thyroid gland are among the most common types of hormonal disorders, and affect large numbers of people. Many of these problems can be helped by administering a synthetic hormone, similar to that produced by the gland. Of the wide range of thyroid disorders, by far the most important are overactivity (hyperthyroidism) and underactivity (hypothyroidism). Both of

◄ *The insert is a section of the thyroid, which clearly shows the cells that produce and store the essential hormone thyroxine.*

▼ *The anatomic drawing shows the position of the thyroid gland in relation to the surrounding structures in the throat, which include the Adam's apple and the trachea.*

blood capillary

cavity filled with colloid in which thyroxine is stored

cells that make thyroxine

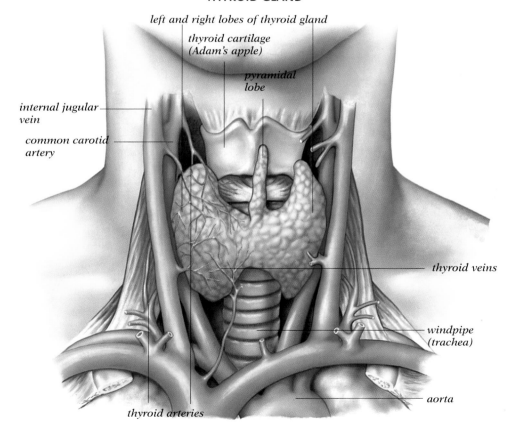

THYROID GLAND

left and right lobes of thyroid gland

thyroid cartilage (Adam's apple)

pyramidal lobe

internal jugular vein

common carotid artery

thyroid veins

windpipe (trachea)

thyroid arteries

aorta

Questions and Answers

Are thyroid problems really so much more common in women than in men?

Yes. Underactivity of the thyroid happens in about 14 in every 1,000 women and only about one in every 1,000 men. Overactivity occurs in at least 20 in every 1,000 women, but in only about one or two in every 1,000 men.

Generally, thyroid disorders are quite common, and more than 3 percent of women are likely to have some type of thyroid problem. Most thryoid disorders can be treated effectively.

I had an overactive thyroid and was treated with pills. Although I have been better for the past two years, the clinic still insists on seeing me. Why is this necessary?

Thyrotoxicosis responds well to treatment with pills. However, the disease does tend to recur, although there may be several years between attacks. It is important to diagnose the disease in the early stages, when it is easier to treat; also, irreversible changes in processes such as the heart rhythm may occur if the disease is allowed to progress too far. For these reasons the doctors will want to keep an eye on you.

Is it true that your hair falls out if you have myxedema?

Myxedema is underactivity of the thyroid gland, and it leads to dry, coarse hair that is very difficult to manage. The disease is also associated with alopecia, in which the hair roots die and the hair falls out. However, this condition is not a direct result of the low thyroid levels.

Do thyroid disorders tend to run in families?

Yes they do, and this is quite common. It is also interesting to note that although one family member might have an overactive thyroid, another person might have an underactive thyroid.

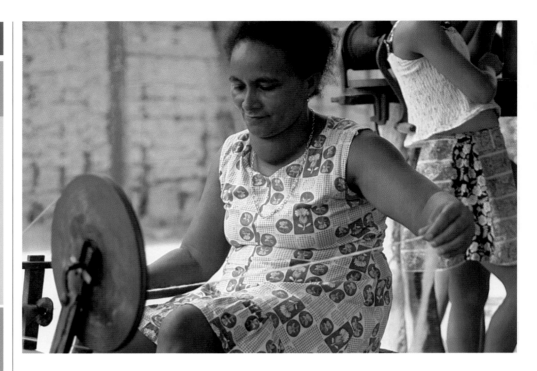

▲ *In some areas of the world, such as the Matto Grosso in Brazil, the normal diet lacks iodine. This deficiency causes the thyroid to malfunction and swell, leading to endemic goiter, the disfiguring condition this woman is suffering from.*

these problems are much more common in women than in men, and up to 2 percent of the adult female population may suffer from an overactive thyroid at some time in life. An underactive thyroid is only slightly less common. Another disorder of the thyroid is thyroiditis, which is an inflammation of the thyroid as a result of a viral infection (see Viruses).

Position and function

The thyroid gland is located in the neck just below the level of the larynx, which can be seen or felt as the Adam's apple. There are two lobes to the gland, and these lie just in front and at either side of the windpipe, or trachea, as it passes down the front of the neck. The two lobes are connected by a small bridge of tissue, and there may be a smaller central lobe called the pyramidal lobe. In an adult the thyroid gland weighs about 0.7 ounce (20 g).

The function of the gland is to produce the thyroid hormone, thyroxine. When the gland is examined under a microscope many small follicles can be seen; these are islands of tissue containing collections of colloid, a protein substance to which the thyroid hormone is bound and from which it can be released under the influence of enzymes. Once thyroxine has been released from the gland into the bloodstream it is taken up by most of the cells of the body. A receptor on the surface of cell nuclei responds to the hormone. The overall effect is to increase the amount of energy that the cell uses; it also increases the amount of protein that the cell manufactures. Although the exact role of the hormone in the cell is not known, it is essential for life. The thyroid gland contains iodine, which is vital for its activity. The thyroid is the only part of the body that requires iodine and it is efficient at trapping available iodine from the blood. An absence of iodine in the diet results in malfunction of the thyroid and growth of the gland; this is endemic goiter.

Control of thyroid activity

The thyroid is one of the endocrine glands under the control of the pituitary gland. The pituitary produces thyroid-stimulating hormone (TSH), which acts on the thyroid to increase the amount of thyroid hormone released. The amount of TSH produced by the pituitary increases if the amount of thyroxine circulating in the system falls, and decreases if it rises. This system, called negative feedback, results in a relatively constant level of thyroid hormone in the blood.

The pituitary gland is controlled by the hypothalamus, and the amount of TSH it produces is increased when TRH (TSH-releasing hormone) is released from the hypothalamus. Most of the

Cancer of the thyroid

PROBLEM	INCIDENCE		TREATMENT
Papillary	The most common type; occurs in young people, including children		By surgery, followed by radioactive iodine treatment if necessary. Outlook is good.
Follicular	Slightly less common; also occurs in young people		As for papillary carcinoma. Outlook is good.
Anaplastic	Uncommon; occurs in the elderly		Surgery is often impossible. X-ray treatment may be used.
Medullary	Very uncommon. Familial.		Surgery. Outlook is good in most cases.

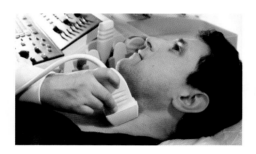

▲ *A radiologist carries out an ultrasound scan of the thyroid.*

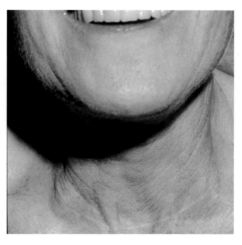

▲ *A thyroidectomy—surgery to remove overactive tissue—may be necessary to combat hyperthyroidism. The scar left by the surgery is insignificant.*

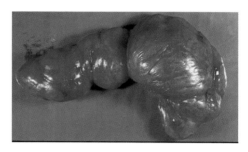

▲ *This is a grossly enlarged thyroid gland that was removed. It measures over 10 in. (25 cm).*

hormone released from the thyroid gland is in the form of tetraiodothyronine, which contains four iodine atoms and is known as T_4. However, the active hormone at the cell level is triiodothyronine, which contains three iodine atoms and is known as T_3. Although the thyroid releases some T_3 into the blood, most of its output is T_4, and this is converted into T_3 in the tissues. Sometimes the tissues switch the way that they convert T_4 to produce an ineffective compound called reverse T_3. As a result, there will be less thyroid hormone activity in the tissues even though the amount of hormone in the bloodstream is adequate (see Hormones).

Any enlargement of the thyroid gland is called goiter. Small but visible goiters are found in about 15 percent of the population, and are about four times more common in women than in men. Usually these are of no significance. In the past, iodine deficiency was the main cause of goiter, but now most goiters are caused by overactivity of the thyroid, or they are simple goiters that are not related to any abnormality of thyroid function. In a few cases, goiters are isolated lumps (nodules) in the substance of the thyroid, and these should be investigated using an ultrasound scan to see whether the lump is composed of functioning tissue. If it is not, and if an ultrasound scan shows that it is solid, then it could be malignant and may need a surgical exploration.

Overactive thyroid glands

Most cases of thyroid overactivity (thyrotoxicosis) are caused by Graves' disease. A goiter is usually present and the eyes become protruding and staring, a sign that many people associate with thyroid problems. It is the basic disease process, and not overactivity, that causes the symptoms (see Symptoms).

Graves' disease is caused by the presence of antibodies in the blood. Although these antibodies do not destroy thyroid tissue, they stimulate the gland to produce thyroid hormone. It is not known why some people are more prone to making these antibodies than others, although there is certainly genetic susceptibility. This can be demonstrated by the fact that many sufferers have a specific type of tissue group.

The effects of an overactive thyroid are: weight loss, increased appetite, anxiety and nervousness (sometimes with a tremor), palpitations of the heart, sweating, intolerance of heat, and irritability. In addition to eye problems, there may be weakness of the muscles, particularly at the shoulders and hips.

Once Graves' disease is suspected, the majority of cases can be diagnosed very simply by measuring the level of thyroid hormone in the blood. Often the T_3 level is measured as well as, or instead of, the T_4 level, since T_3 is always raised in Graves' disease but it is possible to have the disease with a normal T_4 level.

Treatment for Graves' disease is to suppress thyroid activity. This can be done with pills, which must be taken for a year or more. If the gland is very large then it may be appropriate to surgically remove some of it. The alternative is to give a dose of radioactive iodine. This is taken up by the thyroid so it presents no danger to other tissues. It will reduce the level of thyroid activity over the course of approximately six weeks. While the hormone levels are being brought under control, the symptoms can be alleviated by drugs

Thyroid problems			
PROBLEM	**CAUSE**	**EFFECTS**	**TREATMENT**
Simple goiter	Unknown	Swelling of the thyroid, producing a swelling of the neck	Often unnecessary, but in many cases the problem responds to low doses of thyroid hormone pills
Endemic goiter	Lack of iodine in the diet	May lead to deficiency of thyroid hormone	Replacement of iodine in the diet
Myxedema or hypothyroidism	Inadequate levels of thyroid hormone in the blood. May be caused by Hashimoto's disease or autoimmune thyroid failure.	Problem develops slowly, leading to dry rough skin, tiredness, intolerance of cold, increase in weight, constipation, hoarse voice, and deafness	Replacement of thyroid hormone in pill form
Thyrotoxicosis or hyperthyroidism	Most commonly Graves' disease; others include nodules in the thyroid, either single or multiple	Increase in appetite (often with weight loss), sensitivity to heat, disorders of heart rhythm, nervousness, tiredness, and sweating. In some cases there is muscular weakness.	Various treatments, including use of pills, surgery to remove overactive thyroid tissue, and use of radioactive iodine administered by mouth
Graves' disease	Presence of antibodies in the blood, which stimulate the thyroid	Causes thyrotoxicosis; also affects the eyes, causing the pop eyes associated with overactive thyroid	Troublesome eye problems can necessitate surgery, either to tack down the lids to protect the eyes, or to try to reduce the amount of eye protrusion
Thyroiditis	Inflammation of the thyroid gland resulting from a viral infection	Painful swollen gland that may come on suddenly. Mild thyrotoxicosis may result.	Usually unnecessary; painkillers may be given. In severe cases steroid drugs are sometimes used to reduce the inflammation.
Dyshormonogenesis	Inherited abnormality in the way the gland makes hormones. Of six different types the most common is Pendred's syndrome, which is associated with deafness.	A low level of hormone in the blood may cause the same effects as myxedema. There is often a large goiter.	Thyroid hormone
Congenital hypothyroidism (cretinism)	Failure of the fetal thyroid to develop	Mental and physical retardation is the major effect; it occurs in about one in every 4,000 births	Early diagnosis is vital; treatment will help normal development; retardism will otherwise occur

that block the effects of epinephrine, since high levels of thyroid seem to produce an increased response to epinephrine.

Underactive thyroid glands

Underactivity of the thyroid gland (myxedema) results in a lack of thyroid hormone, and a resultant slowing of the body's reactions. One of the most common reasons for hypothyroidism is Hashimoto's disease, in which antibodies in the body appear to damage the thyroid permanently.

In many cases weight gain results, together with a lack of energy, dry thick skin, thinning hair, intolerance of cold, a slow heartbeat, hoarseness, deafness, and a typical puffy face. The presence of hypothyroidism makes elderly people much more susceptible to the condition of hypothermia. Underactivity of the thyroid is readily diagnosed by blood tests. The level of T4 is reduced, but this is not conclusive, since a reduced T4 level can also occur when the thyroid is functioning normally—in severe illness, for example. Much more significant is the high level of TSH that is found in the blood in myxedema, because the pituitary gland tries to stimulate the thyroid to produce enough hormones.

Once a diagnosis is made, the thyroid hormone T4 (thyroxine) can be given by mouth. The dose is built up fairly gradually, since there is a risk of making patients with heart disease worse; myxedema predisposes to coronary artery disease, since it causes a very high level of cholesterol (see Heart Disease).

Patients with myxedema must continue to take medication for the rest of their lives. Although Graves' disease is not quite as easy to treat as myxedema, the results of treatment in both cases is usually satisfactory, and the outlook is very good in both conditions once the early difficulties are overcome.

See also: **Glands; Goiter**

Tinnitus

Commonly described as ringing in the ears, tinnitus is a disturbing condition, in which people hear sounds in one or both ears even though there is no external noise. Although it is an irritating disorder, it is not dangerous.

My son often goes to heavy metal rock concerts where the music is very loud. Will he get tinnitus?

There is every chance that he will get temporary tinnitus—a ringing or high-pitched tone audible only to himself—after going to a very loud rock concert. However, it is unlikely that he will do himself any permanent damage, or get long-term tinnitus, unless he goes every night or joins a band. If he puts his head close to the speakers then he might do himself some permanent harm; but he, or for that matter anybody, is more likely to get tinnitus after being exposed to loud noise every day at places of work. Ear protectors should be worn when anyone comes into contact with prolonged noise. People who shoot for sport must also wear ear protectors, since repeated loud bangs are likely to cause ear damage and tinnitus.

I have tinnitus in one ear only, and although it doesn't worry me too much, my doctor says I should have a checkup once a year. Is this really necessary?

Tinnitus in only one ear, called unilateral tinnitus, is likely to be caused by some disease that might eventually need treatment. Because the cause of your tinnitus may not be obvious at the moment, your doctor is being prudent in ensuring that you are seen every year for a checkup.

I have very loud and unbearable tinnitus and have begged my doctor to remove the hearing apparatus from my ears but he refuses. Why won't he do this?

Because you will learn to live with it. Your doctor is correct in refusing to destroy your ability to hear, as even afterward you might still have the tinnitus. It could even be worse than before.

Tinnitus, the sensation of noise in the ears or head, is a symptom that affects more people than is generally realized. The sound is perceived by the sufferer even though it has no origin outside the body. Although tinnitus is rarely the symptom of any serious disease, it can be extremely disturbing to someone suffering from it. The sound perceived can vary between a ringing, a hissing, a buzzing, and a roaring noise; but the nature and quality of the sound actually have very little to do with the causes. However loud the tinnitus may be, it is always at a lower volume than almost any sound heard from an external source, and a simple comparison with very quiet sounds will show this to be the case. This can be psychologically helpful to a tinnitus sufferer.

The effects of tinnitus vary greatly. In some people the noise is soft and barely noticeable, while in others the noise seems crashingly loud and can prevent the person from sleeping. The cause of this often distressing symptom can arise in any section of a person's hearing apparatus, from the outside of the ear to the intricate neural pathways in the brain (see Hearing).

Outer-ear causes

In the outer ear there are two common causes of tinnitus. The first, and most common, is impacted wax, often caused when people try to clean their ears with cotton swabs, or the corner of a handkerchief. The quick and simple way to remove it is by syringing (see Syringing), in which a doctor washes the wax away with water (see Earwax). The other cause of tinnitus in the external ear is infection by a bacteria or a fungus. If this is the case, the patient complains of both tinnitus and some kind of irritation. Treatment is simple, and antibiotics and steroid drops quickly clear up the infection. After a course of treatment, the tinnitus abates.

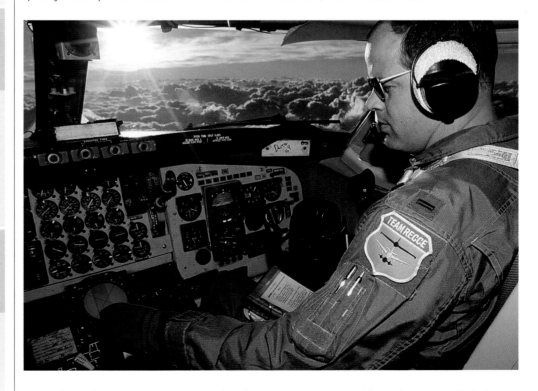

▲ *Prolonged exposure to constant loud noise can cause cochlear damage, which is a cause of tinnitus. Pilots must wear ear protectors to prevent this problem.*

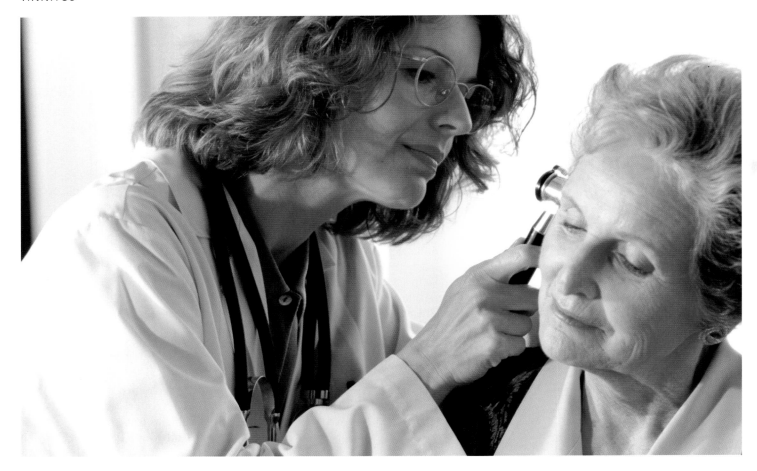

▲ *Using an otoscope, a doctor examines the ear of someone suffering from tinnitus. Hearing tests may also be done, as well as other tests to look for any underlying problem.*

Middle-ear causes

Tinnitus also crops up in association with problems in the middle ear. The two main causes are, first, infection; and, second, otosclerosis.

As with most types of infection, there are acute and chronic conditions. Acute infection of the middle ear, known as acute otitis media (see Otitis), as well as causing tinnitus, can also cause a discharge of mucus from the ear, a raised temperature, and deafness. The best treatment for this is a course of antibiotics and also the use of decongestant nasal drops.

Chronic infection of the middle ear is usually rather more difficult to detect. The symptoms, although broadly similar to those of acute otitis media, are extremely variable and can be intermittent. Rarely, the patient suffers vertigo. If this happens, the patient must seek medical help rapidly to avoid severe and permanent hearing damage (see Vertigo).

Tinnitus is an early symptom of the second type of problem in the middle ear. In this condition, otosclerosis, new bone is deposited around the stirrup bone (stapes) and the deposits prevent the stapes from moving freely and transmitting sound properly from the eardrum to the inner ear. The patient becomes progressively more deaf, but an operation can be performed in which the stapes is removed and a plastic replacement fitted. The surgery restores the hearing, and any remaining tinnitus is usually masked by the increased volume of external sound heard by the patient.

Inner-ear causes

In the inner ear, there are very delicate receptor cells in the cochlea. Damage to receptor cells is by far the most common cause of tinnitus. The damage can have several causes, the most usual of which is the simple degenerative aging process that produces deafness. Although the degree of deafness and the age of onset vary greatly there is almost always some tinnitus (see Deafness). Often, patients complain bitterly about it at night because usually there is no other noise to mask the tinnitus. Another increasingly common cause of tinnitus is cochlear damage caused by sudden loud noises or prolonged exposure to noises of lesser intensity. Where there is loud, constant noise, especially in the workplace in certain occupations, ear protectors should be worn.

Some drugs, when given in high doses, can also cause cochlear damage, and thus tinnitus, and care should always be taken if a drug is likely to produce such a side effect. A disease called Ménière's disease involves tinnitus, and a rare benign tumor, called an acoustic neuroma, can cause tinnitus, usually only in one ear.

Treatment

In general, tinnitus caused by damage to the cochlea can be difficult to treat. Often, a hearing aid that boosts sounds from outside the head will make sufferers less aware of their tinnitus (see Hearing Aids). Devices that appear to mask the sound give some relief, as do relaxant pills. However, the vast majority of people with tinnitus learn to live with the condition.

See also: **Ménière's disease**

Tiredness

Questions and Answers

Do ordinary tonics, bought over the counter, have any value?

Tonics are very much out of fashion these days, but there is no harm in taking them provided that they do not lull you into a false sense of security and become an inadequate substitute for getting proper advice. In effect, no tonic has the near-miraculous properties that may be claimed. If symptoms persist, you must go to your doctor to find out what is really the matter.

What is the difference between laziness and tiredness that is due to illness?

This is not nearly as easy to determine as you might think, so people often mistake one for the other. In general, the lazy person bucks up and finds a huge amount of energy to do what he or she enjoys doing, whereas a truly exhausted person cannot summon up enthusiasm for anything. If in doubt, it is wise to suspect a physical cause until successive negative medical tests make it increasingly unlikely.

My mother, who is 81, seems very feeble and lethargic lately. She thinks this condition is due to her age and won't consult her doctor. Is there anything I can do?

Although there is some loss of energy in old age, it should be slight and gradual. Anything more should not be accepted as normal or inevitable and should be investigated, since it can often be helped. Anemia and inadequate nutrition may be due to a reluctance to buy and cook nutritious food; this is common in old people. Try to persuade your mother to see her doctor about her tiredness; and if necessary make an appointment and take her yourself.

It is perfectly natural to feel really worn out at the end of a hard day at work, after strenuous exercise, or after a few nights' poor sleep. However, tiredness can be one of the first signs of a serious underlying illness.

Tiredness is one of the most common of complaints. Usually, it is short-lived and does not cause concern. However, because it can be the first and sometimes the only indication of something more serious, continuing or persistent tiredness should always be investigated.

Tiredness is often thought to be normal in old age, and certainly there may be a decline in normal vigor (see Aging). In many old people, however, what they may accept as the normal tiredness of aging can sometimes be due to a slowly developing anemia or even an inadequate diet. Tiredness should therefore never be regarded as normal or inevitable until other causes have been ruled out, since many conditions can easily be corrected.

One of the most important features of tiredness due to illness is that it occurs in circumstances when normal tiredness would not be expected. For example, tiredness is normal at the end of the day, after a sleepless night, following severe exertion, in the weeks after an illness or surgery, during pregnancy, or after confinement, whereas tiredness occurring at other times is abnormal, and is likely to be due to disease of some sort. Persistent tiredness should therefore always be investigated, particularly when it is accompanied by symptoms of weakness.

Causes due to illness

Tiredness due to illness may result from either physical or mental disorder, or a combination of the two. Probably the most common physical cause is infection in some part of the body (see

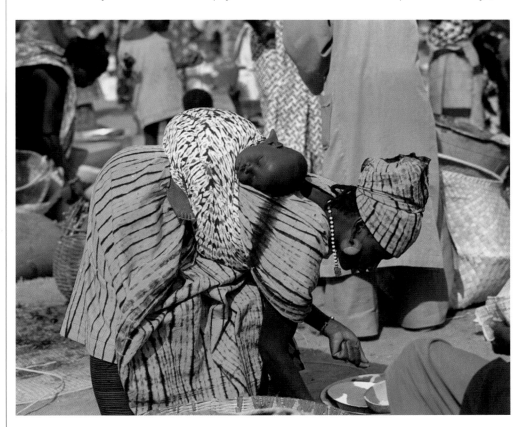

▲ *A tired baby can sleep anywhere, especially when closely bound to his mother. The baby's blissful oblivion blots out all the noise of this vibrant African street market.*

Questions and Answers

I have been feeling tired for some months. Since I am 50 and my periods have stopped, I feel it must be due to the change of life. What can I do about it, and should I be worried if the tiredness does not go away?

You may be right in assuming that your tiredness is due to menopause. On the other hand the tiredness may be completely unrelated to menopause. The danger with tiredness is that we assign reasons so that we don't have to deal with it. Instead we should be getting it properly investigated. So, even though your tiredness may be due to menopause, you should let your doctor investigate to make sure that you do not have another underlying condition that requires treatment. If you have reached menopause, the doctor will be able to prescribe something to lessen its impact on your daily life.

I have been very tired and depressed recently. Is there anything I can do to get rid of this feeling?

Yours is an increasingly common situation these days. It is difficult, in many cases, to know whether someone is suffering from depression or from a physical disease that is primarily responsible for tiredness. The first thing to do is to stand back and consider if there is anything that might be making you depressed. Look, too, for other possible symptoms of physical illness. You could try to put things right yourself for a while by making sure that you get enough sleep and are having an adequate diet, and by sorting out any possible causes of depression. Don't try, however, to carry on for too long on your own without getting medical help. If your tiredness has not improved within four weeks, you must arrange to see your doctor to find out what the problem is and, if something is wrong, to get it sorted out. There are countless people who just struggle on with feelings of tiredness when the cause could be easily removed.

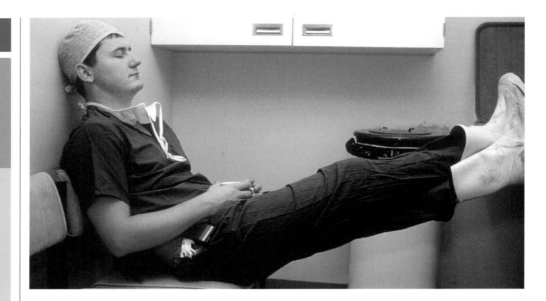

▲ *A tired, overworked doctor is overcome with exhaustion and puts up his feet for a well-earned break.*

Infection and Infectious Diseases), and doctors try to eliminate infection as a cause of persistent tiredness. Established or well-developed infectious diseases such as measles, chicken pox, and influenza (especially if they are accompanied by fever) do make people feel tired and run-down (see Chicken Pox; Influenza; Measles). Tiredness alone may also be an indication that an infection is on the way, for example in the days leading up to flu.

Tiredness that develops or persists for no apparent reason is often due to a localized pocket or focus of infection in some part of the body. A chronic dental, throat, or sinus infection, or a hidden abscess somewhere in the body, is a common cause. Up until the 1950s one of the most likely and most feared causes was a developing tuberculosis infection, in which tiredness was often the only symptom. Tuberculosis is once again resurgent (see Tuberculosis).

Another common cause of persistent tiredness occurring on its own is anemia (see Anemia). Even a slight fall below normal in the level of hemoglobin (the oxygen-carrying compound in the blood) will cause a degree of tiredness and lack of energy. Some hormone disorders may also show themselves primarily in terms of tiredness (see Hormones). The most common of these are

▼ *A combination of late-night studying and perhaps a too warm classroom causes tiredness, and students start yawning and fighting to keep awake.*

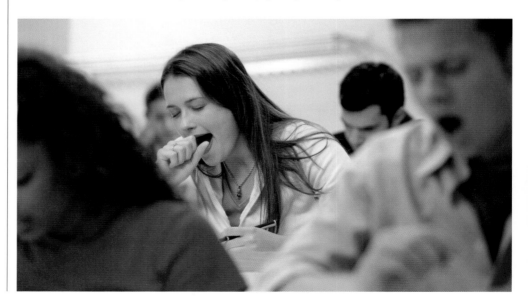

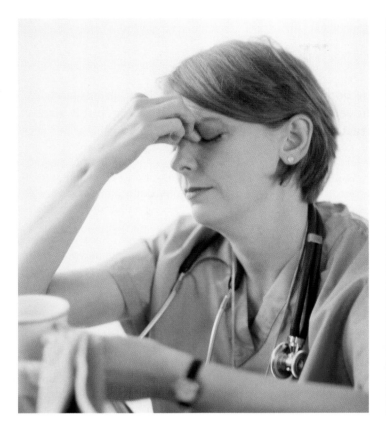

▲ *Long hours on duty can cause extreme tiredness; this doctor is having some caffeine to stave off fatigue.*

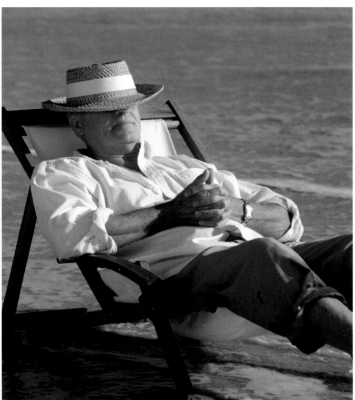

▲ *Sun and sea air can be a very relaxing combination that easily induce tiredness and napping.*

a lack of thyroid hormone, as in someone with an underactive thyroid (myxedema), and lack of insulin, as in diabetes. Another type of metabolic tiredness is obesity (see Obesity). Those who are overweight do, however they may try to disguise it, get tired much more easily than other people. This is partly a direct metabolic effect and partly due to the extra energy used up in carrying additional fat.

An important cause of tiredness, especially in old people, and one that is often unsuspected, is a minor degree of heart failure. This does not mean that the heart has stopped beating, but its pumping action is insufficient to allow even minor exertion. In dilated cardiomyopathy, for instance, a heart chamber may balloon out a little so that it is less able to contract and pump blood. The condition can be greatly helped by recent drugs such as ACE inhibitors.

The underlying disease that doctors are most concerned to rule out in cases of unexplained tiredness is cancer. Tiredness may be the only indication that all is not well with the patient in the early stages of cancer, wherever it is developing. Cancer is sometimes accompanied by a falling off in appetite and a loss of weight as well.

Sometimes the origin of tiredness is due to mental or emotional causes rather than to some physical disease. Boredom, anxiety, and depression make people feel sluggish and dispirited. The sleeplessness that often goes with these conditions will aggravate the tiredness. Anyone with tiredness that does not improve within three or four weeks should see his or her doctor.

Assessing tiredness

In order to assess tiredness and unravel its cause, the doctor has to do several things. He or she will first of all need to have a full account of any symptoms that have been noticed, in order to get a clear idea of its duration, its extent, and the full range of its effects. Because tiredness can be such a vague and variable condition, this is one of the medical situations in which the patient's account of the circumstances, and description of what has been noticed, is particularly important. The doctor's questioning, and the examination that will probably be necessary, will have to cover all the possible causes and may involve virtually any part of the body. From the patient's answers, a doctor will be able to decide what further tests are required.

Treatment

It is unlikely that the doctor will prescribe any medicine until he or she knows the cause of the tiredness. In particular, doctors are very unlikely to give any kind of stimulant drug to relieve tiredness. This can provide only a short-term and artificial boost; it will not address the real problem, and could lead to addiction.

The doctor may suggest adjustments in a patient's lifestyle or diet, and will want to make sure that the patient is getting enough rest and relaxation. The doctor may prescribe a tonic, but the effect of this, apart from possibly stimulating the appetite, is largely a psychological placebo effect.

There is a danger that if a tonic is bought from a drugstore, it could become a dangerous substitute for addressing the problem and getting it properly investigated and treated by a doctor.

> *See also:* **Anxiety; Cancer; Depression; Diabetes; Zest**

Tongue

The tongue is one of the body's muscles, but it is a muscle of an unusual kind. Not only are its movements vital for speaking and eating, but it also contains thousands of taste buds that give us our sense of taste.

The tongue is shaped like a triangle—wide at the base and tapering almost to a point at its tip. It is attached at its base or root to the lower jaw, or mandible, and to the hyoid bone of the skull. At its sides the root is joined to the walls of the pharynx, the cavity that forms the back of the mouth.

The middle part of the tongue has a curved upper surface, and its lower surface is connected to the floor of the mouth by a thin strip of tissue called the frenulum. The tongue's tip is free to move, but when a person is not eating or speaking it normally lies neatly in the mouth with its tip resting against the front teeth.

The sense of taste

The structures that give the tongue its characteristic rough texture are the ridged folds, or papillae, that cover the upper surface of the front two-thirds of the tongue. Largest of these are the eight to 12 V-shaped, or vallate, papillae that form the border between the ridged and unridged areas. Because the papillae are so numerous, they provide a huge surface area to accommodate the 9,000 or more taste buds with which the human tongue is equipped.

This large surface also creates a much increased area on which substances can be dissolved, tested, and tasted. Dissolving is a vital part of the tasting process because the taste buds will not work unless they are presented with molecules in solution. The taste buds nestle in the valleys of the papillae and consist of bundles of hairlike cells, which project into the valley. Nerve fibers

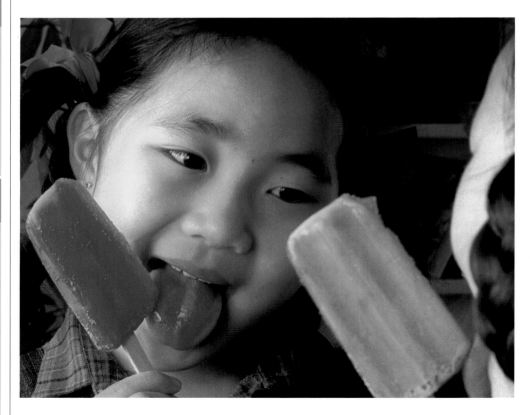

▲ *Licking a Popsicle is a study in contrasting sensations: flavor explodes onto the tongue, while the frostiness lends a biting effervescence to the taste.*

THE TONGUE: ITS POSITION AND STRUCTURE

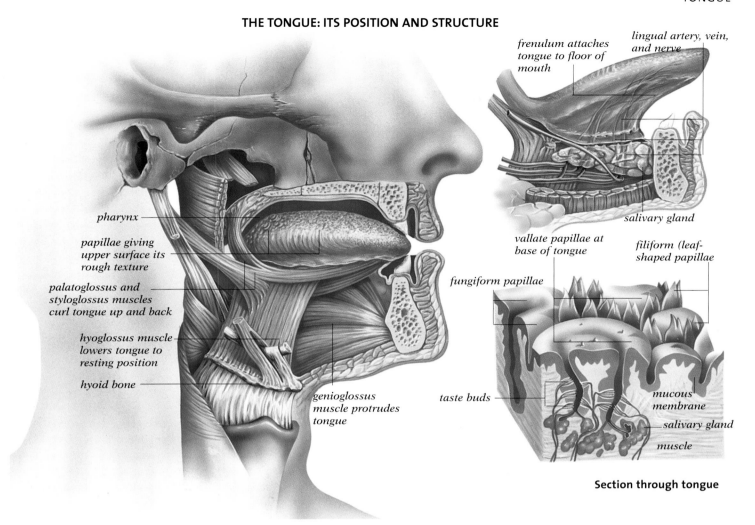

frenulum attaches tongue to floor of mouth

lingual artery, vein, and nerve

pharynx

papillae giving upper surface its rough texture

palatoglossus and styloglossus muscles curl tongue up and back

hyoglossus muscle lowers tongue to resting position

hyoid bone

genioglossus muscle protrudes tongue

salivary gland

vallate papillae at base of tongue

filiform (leaf-shaped papillae

fungiform papillae

taste buds

mucous membrane

salivary gland

muscle

Section through tongue

▲ *These illustrations show the position of the tongue and surrounding musculature (above); the underside, with its blood and nerve supply (top right); and the upper surface with papillae (above right).*

connected to the hair cells run to the brain and to the salivary glands that are situated around the borders of the mouth.

When food is taken into the mouth, nerve cells in the tongue first feel it and test it for texture and temperature. As the taste buds become stimulated by chemical messages arriving from dissolved foodstuff molecules, they send messages to the salivary glands, which pour their secretions into the mouth, not just to help soften the food but also to assist in the dissolving process (see Saliva).

As a result of the combined action of the nerve cells in the tongue, messages are passed to the brain about the taste of food and about its texture and temperature, to give an overall impression of each mouthful (see Nervous System). Because of the tongue's millions of minute undulations, chemicals may be trapped in the valleys for some time, allowing a taste to linger in the mouth long after a mouthful of food or drink has been swallowed.

Movements of the tongue

The actions of the tongue are determined by the muscles it is made up of and to which it is joined, and the way it is fixed in position.

The tongue contains muscle fibers running both longitudinally and from side to side, and these are capable of producing some movement. However, the actions of the tongue are given huge versatility by the contractions of a variety of muscles situated in the neck and at the sides of the jaws. The styloglossus muscle in the neck, for example, is responsible for bringing the tongue upward and backward; the hyoglossus muscle, also located in the neck, brings it back down again into the normal resting position.

In eating, one of the main functions of the tongue is to present the food to the teeth for chewing and to mold softened food into a ball, or bolus, ready for swallowing. These actions are performed by a range of curling and upward and downward movements. When the task has been completed the tongue pushes the bolus into the pharynx at the back of the mouth from where it enters the esophagus and is swallowed into the stomach.

The actions of the tongue are important to human communication through the enunciation of speech (see Speech). The difference between a crisp, clearly spoken "s" sound and the fuzzy tone of a lisped one is, for example, all to do with tongue action. For someone to discover the range of positions the tongue must adopt during speech, he or she says the sounds of the alphabet out loud, then intones common characteristics such as "sh" and "th." There is a precise tongue position for each sound, and that is vital for enunciating consonants in particular.

Injuries and disease

It is easy for the tongue to be accidentally injured, and this often happens when a person bites his or her tongue.

Because it is so richly supplied with blood vessels, the tongue bleeds profusely when injured. If bleeding is severe, the best sort of first aid is to sit the person upright and, with a clean wad of tissue or a folded handkerchief, try to grip the bleeding area between your thumb and forefinger. If the injured person is an adult, and has not sustained severe injuries elsewhere on the body, he or she may be able to apply pressure to the tongue, but in any case a steady pressure should be maintained for about 10 minutes. If an injury is only minor, the injured person can suck an ice cube. Following accidents, the tongue can block the airway. If someone is unconscious after an accident, he or she should be placed in the recovery position, with the chin forward, so that the airway is left clear.

Action of saliva

The tongue is not often prone to disease, mainly because of the antiseptic action of the saliva that bathes it. The most common problems are ulcers (see Ulcers) and a yeast infection *Candida albicans* (see Thrush).

Unless ulcers are very large or painful, or both, the best treatment is to use a proprietary mouthwash or gel, or to suck lozenges formulated to treat the problem. Cancer of the tongue, often due to

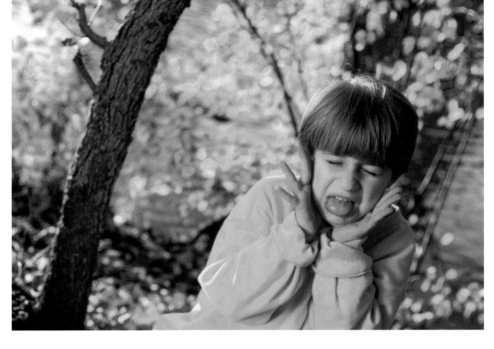

▲ *Sticking out the tongue can be an expression of revulsion or shock, or just an exaggerated reaction to something unpleasant.*

irritation from alcoholic spirits, is fairly common. Cancers of the tongue usually start on the edge of the tongue as a local swelling or ulcer. They can spread widely, so it is vital that people see their doctor if they notice any abnormal swelling or pain in the tongue, or if they have persistent ulcers that do not clear up quickly.

The color, texture, and general state of the tongue can arouse a doctor's suspicions about disease, but the tongue rarely tells the whole story on its own. Normally, the ridged papillae are cleared of debris that accumulates on the tongue by the washing process, which is affected jointly by the saliva and the movements of the tongue.

If a coating of fur does build up on the tongue, it is usually because the flow of saliva is impaired. This may be due to thirst or because a person's appetite is reduced or impaired for some reason, such as a digestive upset, but it could also stem from a psychological problem.

Early treatment

If anyone has persistent discoloration or pain, he or she should always bring this to the attention of the doctor. As is the case with so many disorders, the sooner treatment can begin, the better the chances of a total recovery.

▼ *To examine the throat, sometimes it is necessary to hold the tongue down with a implement called a tongue depressor.*

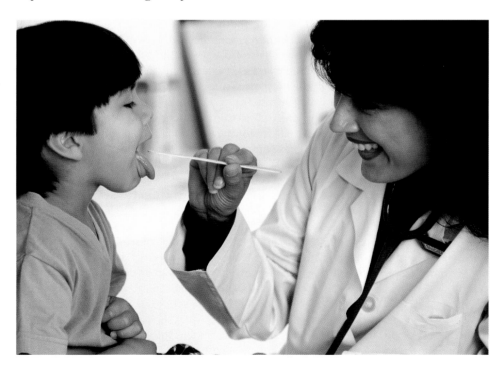

See also: **Body piercing; Cancer; Mouth; Pain; Sores; Speech therapy**

Tonsils

How soon after having an attack of tonsillitis is it safe to have surgery to remove the tonsils?

Two to three weeks is the accepted period, after which time the risk of abnormal bleeding after surgery returns to normal. If a child is having attacks of tonsillitis every 10 days and is due for a tonsillectomy, the doctor will put him or her on a course of antibiotics for three weeks before surgery. This eliminates the possibility of the child's being sent home when he or she is taken to the hospital for surgery.

Should I suck or swallow aspirin when I have a sore throat?

Sucking aspirin can be dangerous, because it can cause a chemical burn on the mucous membranes lining the mouth and the throat.

Will I be more prone to infections after I have had my tonsils out?

No. Your tonsils probably have a significant function only during the first few years of life. That is one of the reasons why doctors prefer not to remove the tonsils of a very young child.

My three-year-old son has very frequent attacks of tonsillitis, but the surgeon is reluctant to remove his tonsils. Why is this?

At three years of age your son will probably weigh between 26 and 40 lb. (12 to 18 kg) and therefore his total blood volume will be between 2 and 3 pt. (950 and 1400 ml). A loss of 0.3 pt. (120 ml), which is the average loss for the operation, would deprive him of between 8 and 12 percent of his blood and cause significant anemia. If he should bleed heavily after the operation his condition would become very serious indeed.

The tonsils have an important role as part of the body's defense system. Viruses and bacteria, however, can cause the tonsils to become inflamed and painful. Recurrent infections may make removal of the tonsils necessary.

The tonsils are part of a ring of lymphoid tissue (Waldeyer's ring) that encircles the entrance to the food and air passages in the throat (see Lymphatic System). Although the tonsils are present at birth they are relatively small. They grow rapidly during the first few years of life, only to regress after puberty. However, they do not disappear completely.

◄▼ *The tonsils encircle the entrance to the food and air passages, in their role of defense against infection. But when the tonsils are infected—and the most common infection is tonsillitis—they become swollen and inflamed, making swallowing, and sometimes breathing, difficult and painful.*

POSITION OF TONSILS

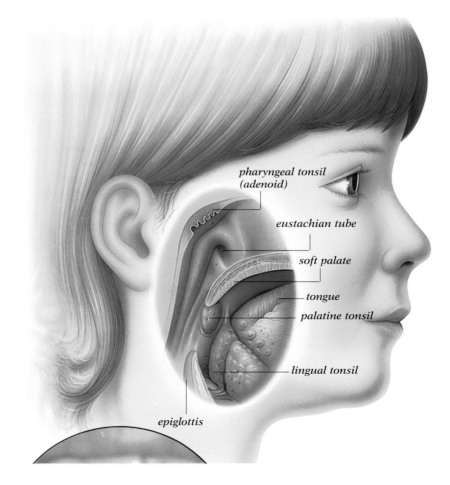

pharyngeal tonsil (adenoid)

eustachian tube

soft palate

tongue

palatine tonsil

lingual tonsil

epiglottis

Questions and Answers

My husband is going into the hospital for a tonsillectomy. How long will he have to stay off work and how should I look after him ?

Most adult patients take about two weeks to recover completely. This includes one week in the hospital and at least one week resting at home. It is important that you encourage your husband to eat as abrasive a diet as he can tolerate so that the site of the operation is kept clean. If it was your child who was having surgery, the recommendation would be the same, with the additional precaution that he or she should not come into contact with other children for a week.

If a person's tonsils are larger than normal, should they be removed?

The size of the tonsils alone rarely necessitates their removal. However, in a few cases the tonsils are so enlarged that they obstruct the passage of air and a tonsillectomy must be performed. The obstruction occurs mainly at night. While the person is asleep he or she stops breathing intermittently and therefore wakes up. The consequence of this condition is called sleep apnea. Subjects may become lethargic, undergo personality changes, and become incontinent. Very rarely, the chronic deprivation of oxygen can lead to heart failure and irregularities of the heart rate.

Is it true that some children have to have their tonsils removed to stop them from going deaf?

Yes. In children, attacks of tonsillitis may precipitate attacks of otitis media (an infection of the middle ear) or may prevent a complete recovery from secretory otitis media, a condition known more commonly as glue ear. In these cases the surgeon may advise tonsillectomy to prevent possible damage to the middle ear and avoid the deafness which, although temporary, is associated with these conditions.

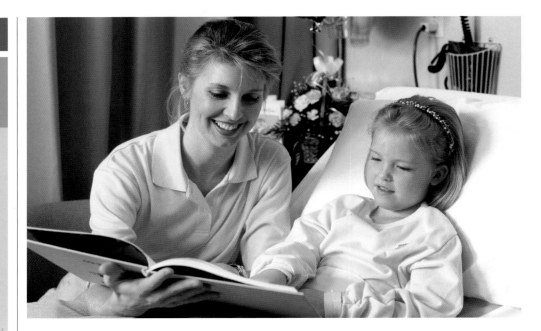

▲ *Although children recover very quickly from a tonsillectomy, being in the hospital can be a lonely experience. The reassuring presence of a parent, especially just before and after surgery, helps speed recovery.*

Function

In childhood, the tonsils are an important part of the immune system and play a significant role in the body's defense mechanisms (see Immune System). They are ideally situated to monitor ingested material and to react to those materials that could pose a threat to the well-being of the body. The tonsils provide immunity against upper respiratory tract infections by producing lymphocytes (see Lymphocytes). In addition, the tonsils produce antibodies that deal with infections locally.

Tonsillitis

Almost everyone suffers an attack of tonsillitis at some time in life. The organism causing the infection is sometimes a dangerous bacterium called streptococcus (see Bacteria).

It is usually easy to distinguish tonsillitis from a simple sore throat because tonsillitis lasts considerably longer—approximately one week. Symptoms vary depending on the severity of the infection, but they always include marked discomfort in the pharynx (see Pharynx), which makes swallowing painful. Pain from the throat may also be felt in the ears. Some patients also experience discomfort on turning their head because of swelling of the glands in this region.

A fever almost always accompanies the infection, but it varies in degree. Children, for example, tend to develop higher temperatures and consequently more symptoms (such as malaise and vomiting) than adults (see Temperature). Some children may have no symptoms in the throat, but will complain of abdominal pain instead.

When the tonsils are infected they become enlarged and inflamed. Specks of pus (see Pus) exude from their surfaces. The infection responds well to antibiotics, and improvement can be expected within 36–48 hours (see Antibiotics). Symptoms can be alleviated by eating soft foods and drinking plenty of liquids. Painkillers such as aspirin both relieve the pain and reduce the temperature (see Aspirin and Analgesics). Aspirin is not recommended for children under the age of 16 as there is a very slight risk of a disorder called Reye's syndrome (see Reye's Syndrome).

Tonsillitis tends to occur most frequently between the ages of four and six years, and then again around puberty. The more often the tonsils are infected, the more prone they are to persistent and recurrent infection. A stage is reached when removal of the tonsils is the only sensible way of controlling the illness.

In some cases an infection is so severe that an abscess forms in the tissue around the tonsils (see Abscess). This is called peritonsillar abscess, or quinsy. Quinsy usually affects one side of the tonsils and is very rare in children. The affected tonsil swells to a considerable extent, and may

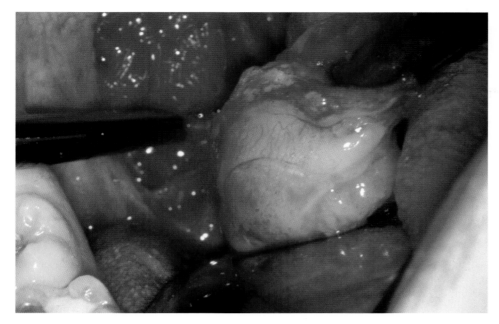

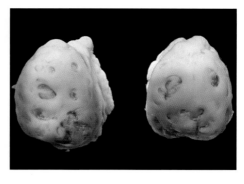

▲ *These tonsils that have been removed show patches of scar tissue from repeated bouts of tonsillitis.*

◄ *Only as a last resort will a person's tonsils be removed. They are dissected from the pharyngeal wall while the patient is under general anesthesia.*

prevent swallowing altogether. Local inflammation contributes to this by limiting the opening of the jaw. Oral antibiotics are not only difficult to swallow but also rarely effective. Higher doses of antibiotics are given by intramuscular injections for 24–36 hours, followed by oral antibiotics. If the quinsy is ripe—that is, the abscess is pointing—recovery may be accelerated by lancing the abscess and allowing the pus to drain.

In exceptional cases, an infection is not limited to the tonsils, but spreads both down the neck to the chest and up toward the base of the skull; this is a parapharyngeal abscess. This is a life-threatening condition and requires urgent admission to the hospital, where the abscess can be drained and treated with massive doses of powerful antibiotics. Patients who have had quinsy are thought to be more susceptible to this complication and are therefore advised to have their tonsils out even if they have not been troubled previously by recurrent tonsillitis.

Viral infections of the tonsils

Tonsillar tissue can be affected by viral infections, which commonly lead to a sore throat. Symptoms are similar to those of tonsillitis, but are milder and last for only 24–48 hours.

The tonsils are also affected in infectious mononucleosis (see Infectious Mononucleosis), in which a sore throat is accompanied by severe lassitude, joint pains, and generalized swelling of all the lymph nodes. In this condition, the tonsils may be covered by a white membrane, and the adjacent palate is dotted with splinterlike hemorrhages. Neither of these conditions is an indication that a tonsillectomy is necessary, since both occur just as frequently in people who have had surgery to remove their tonsils for a variety of other reasons.

Tonsillectomy

A tonsillectomy is performed under general anesthesia. The tonsils are dissected away from the pharyngeal wall and the resulting bleeding is controlled by ligatures. On average about ⅓ pint (120 ml) of blood is lost during surgery, irrespective of the age of a patient. Surgeons are therefore very reluctant to operate on children who are very small or below the age of four, since this amount of blood loss is a significant proportion of their total blood volume. If surgery is necessary, however, a child will be given an intravenous infusion for about 12 hours after the tonsillectomy.

The only serious complication that may occur after a tonsillectomy is further hemorrhage. When this occurs it is usually within the first hours after surgery and requires a return to the operating room for further ligation (see Hemorrhage).

Bleeding may also occur six to ten days after surgery if the tonsil bed becomes infected. Patients most commonly affected are those who eat poorly postoperatively or who have had an attack of tonsillitis immediately before admission to the hospital. Delayed bleeding is treated with antibiotics, but if the patient has lost a lot of blood a transfusion or a course of iron tablets may be necessary to stimulate rapid replacement of the lost blood. Children tend to recover from surgery more quickly than adults and require only one or two days in the hospital. Adults, however, may need to be in the hospital for four to five days until they are fit to be discharged.

Tumors of the tonsils

Tumors of the tonsils are uncommon but may occur at any age. Lymphomas may cause a sudden tonsillar enlargement and are usually associated with swollen glands in other parts of the body—for example, under the arms and in the groin. They generally respond well to treatment, and many patients are cured (see Lymphoma; Tumors). Another type of tumor is known as squamous cell carcinoma. It occurs in the older age group and men are more frequently affected than women. The condition results in a unilaterally enlarged and painful tonsil, which may be ulcerated. Variable degrees of difficulty and pain on swallowing are experienced, and in advanced cases it may even be impossible for the patient to swallow his or her saliva. Similarly, as the disease progresses, the tumor spreads to the glands in the neck. With early treatment a recovery rate of at least 50 percent can be expected.

See also: **Fevers; Painkillers; Streptococcus; Vomiting**

Total allergy syndrome

Everyone knows someone who is allergic to something, but the term "total allergy syndrome" was coined to describe an allergic response to all substances. Does this condition really exist, or is the term a misnomer?

People with what has been called total allergy syndrome seem to become severely ill when exposed to any of a wide range of substances in their environment.

All types of allergic disease are a result of a defect in the body's immune system. When a substance recognized as foreign enters the body, it provokes the production of substances called antibodies. When the foreign substance enters the body again, the antibodies bind to the intruder, rendering the body immune. Some people develop a hypersensitivity to some foreign substances, and the binding of antibody to intruder may inappropriately trigger the release of a number of other chemicals concerned with the defense of the body. The chemicals produce unpleasant effects such as asthma, runny nose, skin rashes, and vomiting (see Immune System).

Most people with an allergic predisposition become sensitized to just one or two substances, and their symptoms on reexposure are generally mild. In more severe cases of allergy, however, not only are the symptoms more alarming, with joint pains and bleeding from the large intestine, but people may become sensitive to a variety of substances, particularly foods.

However, some symptoms in the so-called total allergy syndrome are not likely to happen as a result of immune disorders. In particular, allergy does not make people lose consciousness, although it may certainly cause headaches and a disabling sense of ill health (see Headache; Joints; Unconsciousness).

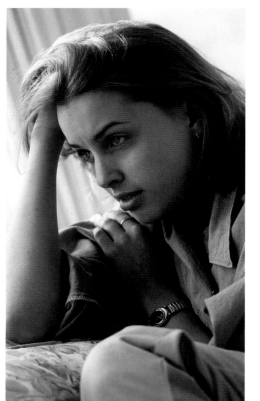

▲ *Whether it exists or not, if people perceive that they suffer from total allergy syndrome, they can experience a variety of symptoms.*

It is true that there is a wide range of substances to which allergy can develop but this does not justify the assumption that many symptoms people suffer are of allergic origin. In particular, the possible significance of foodstuffs or food additives as allergens has been exaggerated, and assertions that food allergies are common have often been made on insufficient grounds. It is not surprising that some people may suffer from the stress of the situation, with the result that anxiety symptoms occur that are not directly related to any action of the immune system (see Anxiety; Psychosomatic Problems).

Treatment

It is difficult to help people whose disease has made such an impact on their lives that they are thought to suffer from total allergy syndrome. It does such people no favor to accept uncritically that they are suffering from an alleged condition that in fact does not exist. To do so is to deny them proper investigation, an accurate diagnosis, and effective treatment.

See also: Allergies; Asthma; Diagnosis; Laboratory tests; Nose; Rashes; Symptoms; Vomiting

Touch

Questions and Answers

Why do babies touch as well as look at everything around them?

Babies train their brain to match the sight of an object with its feel. When they are older, these earlier experiences enable them to predict what the texture of an object or surface is without touching it.

When someone is paralyzed down one side from a stroke, does he or she lose the sense of touch on that side?

Not necessarily. Some people who have been paralyzed by a stroke retain their sense of touch on that side, if the damage has been confined to the parts of the brain that control movement. If the area of damage is sufficiently large to have involved the touch analyzers in the brain or their connections, then the sense of touch will be damaged.

On very cold days my sense of touch is poor. Why?

In cold weather, two things are working against the touch receptors just below the skin in the fingers. The cold itself reduces their efficiency, and blood is diverted away from the skin in order to minimize heat loss; this poor blood supply further impairs the ability of these nerve endings to send concise messages to your brain.

Do blind people have a better sense of touch than the sighted?

Blind people have the same equipment in their nervous system for touch perception. What makes them able to use it more effectively than sighted people is the practice that this sense has had in the absence of sight. The brain has to rely much more on touch, so the analysis of touch has become more efficient, enabling, for example, the rapid reading of braille.

Touch is so fundamental to life that most people never think of how the many sensations they feel are produced: how, for instance, people can tell silk from sandpaper, or recognize an object simply by the way it feels on the skin.

Touch is one of the first ways in which young babies explore their world, and it remains people's most intimate way of relating to their environment. People have a wide range of receptors in their skin that are sensitive to different types of pressure. Through these they are constantly able to monitor their immediate surroundings and keep the brain in touch with the surfaces on which they sit, the objects they grasp, and so on. However, the sensation of touch is complex and is therefore sensitive to disturbances in many parts of the nervous system.

The sensory receptors

Just below the surface of the skin there are many nerve endings with varying degrees of sensitivity. These allow the nervous system to be supplied with different types of touch sensations (see Skin and Skin Diseases).

Wrapped around the base of the fine hairs of the skin are the free nerve endings, which respond to any stimulation of the hair. These touch receptors are the least sophisticated in structure and rapidly stop firing if the hair continues to be stimulated. Receptors found in greater numbers in the hairless part of the skin—for example, on the fingertips and lips—are formed into tiny disks. Because the nerve fibers are embedded within these disks they respond more slowly to pressure and continue to fire when the pressure is maintained. Other more structurally complicated receptors are formed by many membranes wrapped around a nerve ending like an onion skin, and give responses to more constant pressure. In addition, the information that all receptors send into the nervous system tends to be influenced by the temperature at which they are operating. This explains why people's sense of touch can be impaired in cold weather.

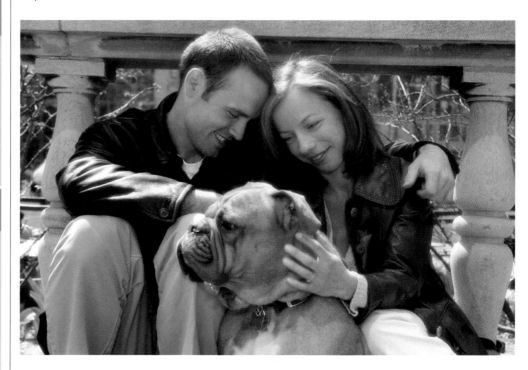

▲ *The sense of touch is an important method of communication in relationships, not only between people, but also between people and animals.*

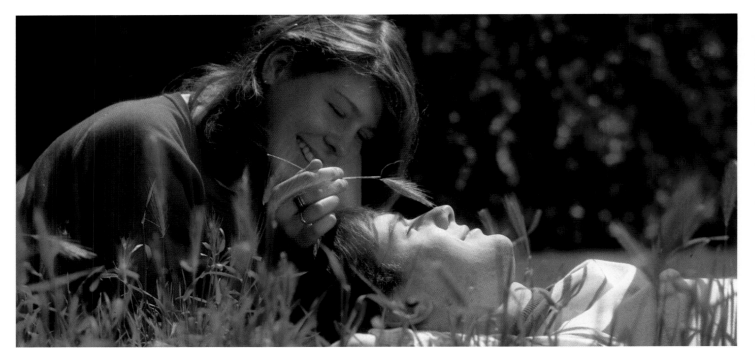

TOUCH PATHWAYS

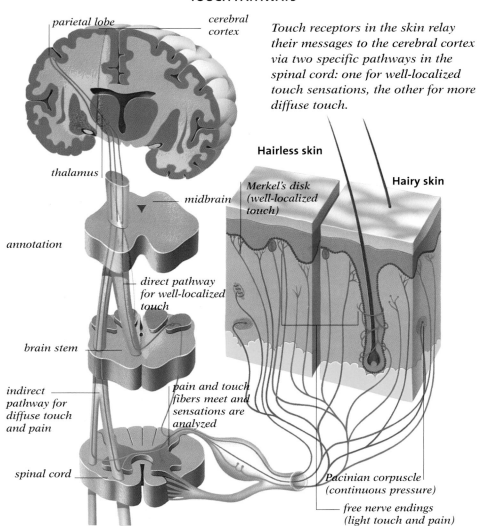

Touch receptors in the skin relay their messages to the cerebral cortex via two specific pathways in the spinal cord: one for well-localized touch sensations, the other for more diffuse touch.

▲ *The touch receptors in our skin are so sensitive that they respond to the gentlest stroking of a blade of grass.*

The distribution of the different types of touch receptors reflects their particular job. The receptors around the base of body hair send messages from large areas of the skin about the pressure stimulating them. They rapidly stop their flow of information once a person has been warned of the presence of an object—for example, an insect on the skin. On the hairless skin, more sophisticated receptors give continuous information, allowing objects to be felt as the brain gathers this information into a coherent picture.

Analysis in the spinal cord

Some of the fibers that convey touch information pass into the spinal cord and, without stopping, go straight up to the brain stem. These fibers deal mainly with sensations of pressure, particularly a specific point of pressure. Therefore, they need to send their messages directly to the higher centers of the brain so that this well-localized sensation can be assessed without confusion from any analysis in the spinal cord.

Other nerve fibers bringing information of more diffuse touch enter the gray matter of the spinal cord and there meet a network of cells that perform an initial analysis of their information. This is the same area that receives messages from the pain receptors in the skin and elsewhere. The meeting in the

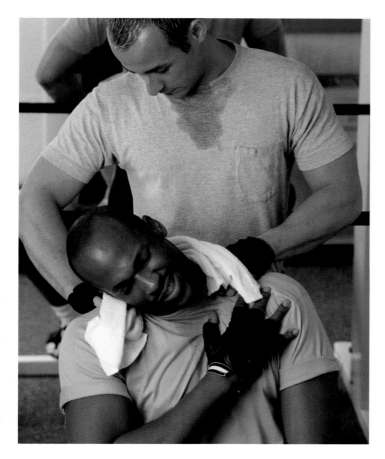

▲ *Touch can physically benefit the body. A massage after strenuous exercise can help to ease muscle aches and pains.*

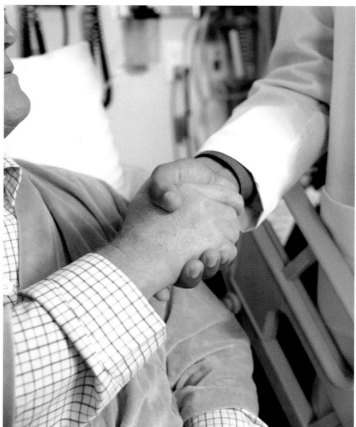

▲ *Touch is often a way of showing friendliness, as in the handshake—a common gesture used to greet people.*

spinal cord of messages dealing with both touch and pain allows for the mixture of these two sensations, and explains such responses as the relief of painful stimuli by rubbing.

This spinal cord analysis filters the sensations, which are then sent upward to the brain. The gray matter of the spinal cord here acts as an electronic gate so that pain information can be suppressed by the advent into the cord of certain types of touch impulse, limiting the amount of trivial information that needs to be transmitted to the higher centers.

This division of the touch pathways to the brain into two streams—one of which goes fairly directly up to the brain stem, and the other that is first analyzed by the cells of the spinal cord—enables the fine discriminating aspects of touch to be preserved. As a result, a person can estimate accurately the amount of pressure in a touch and its position, but if the pressure is too great, or too sharp, the pain analyzers become involved through the connections in the spinal cord and tell the person that the touch is painful as well (see Pain; Pain Management).

The sensory sorting house

Whether touch sensations from the skin have come by the more direct route or after analysis in the spinal cord, they eventually end in the compact knot of gray matter deep in the center of the brain, called the thalamus.

The direct touch fibers will have already relayed once in the brain stem and then will have crossed over to the other side, streaming to the thalamus in a compact bundle. The other fibers will have crossed over to the opposite side of the spinal cord after their relay in the gray matter there; so all the touch sensations from one side of the body are analyzed by the opposite side of the brain.

In the thalamus, these pieces of information from various different types of receptor in the skin are assembled and coordinated. This enables the brain's highest centers in the cerebral cortex to put together a picture of the sensations of touch of which a person becomes conscious.

The final analysis

The area of the brain that enables the complex array of touch sensations entering the nervous system to be consciously perceived is the middle section of the cerebral cortex. As with all other sensory information, touch is analyzed by the cortex in a series of steps, each increasing the complexity of the sensory perception. From the thalamus, the raw data are projected to a narrow strip in the front of the parietal lobes.

This primary sensory area of the cortex processes the information before relaying it to the secondary and tertiary sensory areas. In these latter areas the full picture of the site, type, and significance of the touch sensations a person feels is produced and correlated, along with memories of previous sensations and sensory stimuli coming via the ears and eyes. The latter coordination is achieved easily because the areas for vision and hearing back onto the areas for touch.

Touch sensations are also coordinated in the secondary and tertiary sensory areas with the sensations of what position the limbs, joints, and digits are in. This is vitally important, as it enables people to determine an object's size and shape, and helps them to distinguish one object from another.

Problems

Damage to the nervous system at many different levels can alter a person's ability to feel and notice things that touch his or her skin. How this affects the person depends largely on the exact place in the nervous system that the damage occurs.

Damage to the peripheral nerves, which may happen in alcoholism or in diabetes, for example, can affect the sense of touch (see Alcoholism; Diabetes). However, it takes extensive damage for the sense of touch to be lost completely or severely diminished.

Often people with such disorders feel pins and needles in their hands and feet for some time before any alteration in their sense of touch (see Pins and Needles). The ability of the fingers to make fine touch discrimination may be involved, and sufferers may report feeling as if they have gloves on all the time. Instead of being lost or diminished, the sense of touch can also become distorted as a result of damage to the peripheral nerves, so that a sufferer may say that smooth surfaces feel like sandpaper or warm surfaces feel hot.

Much greater distortion of the sense of touch, however, arises from disease in the spinal cord, for example in multiple sclerosis. The cross connections that arise in the spinal cord if it is diseased, or even pressed upon from the outside, produce distortions of touch that can be disabling and unpleasant. Apart from noticing a feeling

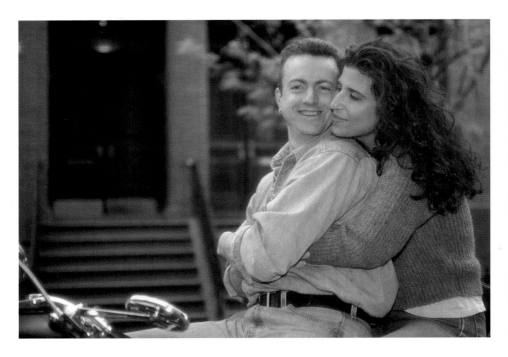

▲ *People tend to show their affection for each other through touch. Hugging, for example, is felt as a pleasant sensation by babies and children as well as adults.*

of numbness, the hands may have lost their ability to make properly coordinated touch perception, for example, in picking the correct coin from a pocket, or the feet may feel as if they are walking on cotton balls instead of firm ground (see Multiple Sclerosis).

Similar types of symptoms can arise from damage to the same touch pathways through the brain stem all the way to the thalamus. Thalamic damage, which happens after strokes, for example, can produce bizarre alterations of touch so that a simple pinprick produces unpleasant, spreading, electric shocklike sensations, or the gentle stroking of a finger may be felt as an unpleasant burning spreading over the skin (see Stroke).

Damage to the parietal lobes of the cerebral cortex, common in strokes and tumors of the brain, may disrupt touch sensations in other ways. If the thalamus is still intact (it is often involved in the disease as well), then the touch will be felt, but the localization of the touch will be inaccurate—it may, for example, be felt on the other side of the body. If the parietal lobe is not functioning, the correlation of different types of sensation will not occur. For instance, usually, when the hand or skin is drawn upon, a person will be able to distinguish letters and numbers, but someone with parietal lobe damage will not recognize shapes, although he or she will be aware that a touch has occurred (see Brain Damage and Disease).

▼ *Touch can help us to discern shapes, so it is obviously important to someone who is blind, since the ability to define shapes is fundamental to reading braille.*

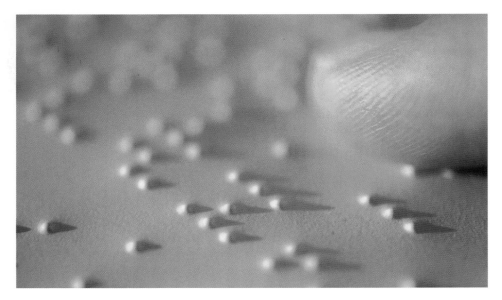

See also: **Brain; Nervous system; Numbness; Spinal cord**

Tourette's syndrome

Questions and Answers

My husband and I have been arguing about Tourette's syndrome. He says it is a new disease; I have no idea, but argue that very few diseases are new and so this one is probably not. Who is right?

A case was described in 1825 but the first full account of the condition, including vocal utterances, was published by the French physician George Gilles de Tourette in 1885. There is every reason to suppose that the disorder existed long before the start of the 19th century but was simply dismissed as a form of temporary insanity. You can fairly claim to have won this argument.

My five-year-old son has developed a very obvious tic in which he turns down the corner of his mouth and tightens a muscle in his neck. I am seriously concerned that he may be developing Tourette's syndrome, especially as one of his uncles had it. Is this likely?

No. Tics in young children, especially boys, are very common while Tourette's syndrome is very rare. In the great majority of cases, childhood tics disappear spontaneously before the end of adolescence. Even if there were a genetic element in this case, the chances of your son's developing the full clinical picture of Tourette's syndrome are small.

Can Tourette's syndrome, or the tendency to develop it, be diagnosed before birth?

No. Doctors are not certain of the cause of this condition and it seems unlikely to be caused by a single gene mutation that could be detected by DNA analysis. Possibly with further advances in genetics it may be possible to demonstrate a tendency, but this is certainly not possible today.

This extraordinary and distressing condition is rare, but for the sufferer and his or her family it can cause embarrassment. In most cases the disorder runs in the family but it is not thought to be wholly genetic; rather it is thought to be caused by a combination of factors, of which genetics is one.

Tourette's syndrome, which affects males four times as often as females, usually begins between the ages of five and about 12. It starts with simple tics—involuntary and apparently uncontrollable body movements such as twitches, shrugs, strong eye closures, or jerks of the shoulders. Tics of this kind are very common in children, especially boys, and will normally have disappeared before the end of the teens (see Twitches and Tics).

Symptoms

In Tourette's syndrome, however, these tics are progressive. Regular childhood tics become more severe and extend to involve multiple twitchings, mainly of the face, neck, and shoulders; grimacing; nodding; sniffing; stuttering; or apparently purposeful body movements often of a grotesque character. For a time, the symptoms are confined to movement defects only, and often the condition never progresses beyond this stage. But in more severe cases the sufferer begins to make noises. Initially these may be simple grunts or cough-like sounds, and, again, the disorder may go no further. But often these effects increase so that grunting, yelping, squealing,

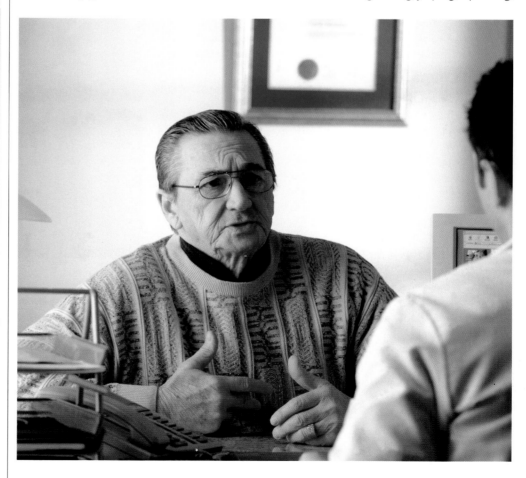

▲ *Describing the symptoms of Tourette's syndrome, even to a doctor, can be very embarrassing, and, for this reason, some patients prefer not to seek any treatment.*

and barking become common occurrences. In the worst case, the affected person develops a compulsive necessity to utter obscene words or remarks. This is called coprolalia and it occurs in about half the cases of the syndrome, so that the condition becomes a severe social liability. Coprolalia may be associated with obscene gestures (copropraxia). Symptoms are often preceded by what is called a sensory urge—a strong feeling that relief from discomfort or tension will be experienced by giving way to the urge to let go and allow the movement or utterance. Sometimes, the syndrome features an involuntary compulsion to imitate the movements of others (echopraxia) or to repeat their words (echolalia).

The distress and embarrassment to the sufferer of these attention-provoking symptoms may be extreme and can often lead to severe social disablement. The awareness of the effect of these symptoms on other people adds to the emotional stress of the affected person and can exacerbate the condition. Once fully established, Tourette's syndrome is usually permanent, but in about one case in 20 there is a full spontaneous recovery.

Diagnosis and associations

Diagnosis is usually obvious from the symptoms and from the fact that they are apparently uncontrollable by the sufferer. Symptoms may differ in different physical situations. They may, for instance, be more severe in church than at home. Initially, there may be some measure of control but this will usually be lost. The degree of severity varies greatly from case to case. Tourette's syndrome has obsessive-compulsive features and may be associated with the other elements of obsessive-compulsive disorder or with another that is fairly common in children, that is, attention deficit hyperactivity disorder.

Causes

It is unlikely that there is a single cause for Tourette's syndrome. In a high proportion of cases there is a known family history. There are also likely to be environmental causal factors.

A temporary lack of oxygen during birth has been proposed as a possible factor. The site of the brain damage is thought to be in the large masses of nerve cells at the base of the brain known as the basal ganglia. These are concerned, among other things, with emotional processes, and it is in these areas that the drugs act that are used to control the symptoms. Symptoms similar to those of Tourette's syndrome occur in a brain disorder called encephalitis lethargica which affects the basal ganglia. Echopraxia and echolalia often occur in encephalitis lethargica.

So far as any genetic cause is concerned, current thought is that the most likely pattern is of a multi-gene dominant disorder with what is called variable penetrance. The idea of variable penetrance actually explains nothing. It is simply a way of commenting on the fact that many dominant gene mutations known to cause a particular disorder do so in less than 100 percent of cases. This is called incomplete penetrance, and in Tourette's syndrome penetrance is thought to vary from case to case. Why this should be true is not known.

Treatment

Many cases of Tourette's syndrome are never treated. This is partly because they are too mild to justify treatment but mainly because of embarrassment and dislike of discussing the problem and because of the assumption that the condition is beyond treatment.

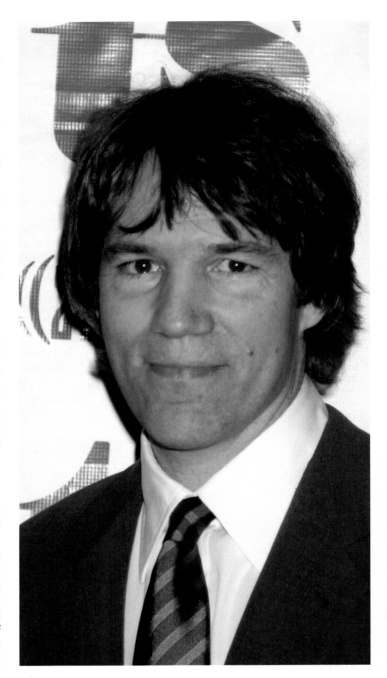

▲ *The Hollywood producer David E. Kelley was honored at the Tourette's syndrome awards dinner. The dinner aims at creating greater public awareness, and generates financial support to fight the disorder.*

Treatment is certainly difficult but claims have been made for the effectiveness of behavior therapy, even in severe cases. Some psychiatrists find tranquilizing drugs helpful, but the most frequently used medications are drugs in the class of antipsychotic drugs known as neuroleptics. These cause emotional quieting, promote indifference, and slow down bodily and mental overactivity. A drug called haloperidol (Serenace) is often used.

See also: **Attention deficit hyperactivity disorder**

Tourniquet

Questions and Answers

How long is it safe to leave a tourniquet on a limb?

The time varies depending on the nature of the tourniquet. Damage can result from pressure on the nerves, and from the limb's being deprived of blood for too long. For these reasons, a tourniquet should be released every 20 minutes, and it should not be left on for more than an hour. When it is first applied, a label with the time written on it should be affixed to the patient prominently so that it is clear when the tourniquet must be loosened.

My son cut his hand and by the time I brought him to the hospital he had lost a lot of blood. Should I have used a tourniquet?

No. You probably could have stopped the bleeding by holding his hand above his head and pressing on the bleeding point with a pad. A tourniquet applied by an inexperienced person is likely to cause unnecessary injury.

When I had a blood test at the hospital, the doctor put a tourniquet on my arm. Was it a tourniquet used in emergencies?

No. You had a venous tourniquet, which exerted only enough pressure to obstruct the flow of blood in the veins, so that the arteries carried on pumping blood into the arm. This enlarged the veins, so the doctor could easily insert a needle to obtain blood.

What is the best thing to use for an emergency tourniquet?

A piece of material that can be tied around the limb may be used. It must not be stretchable, and must be reasonably wide so that it does not cause injury to the limb. A piece of cutlery, such as a spoon, may be used to twist it tight.

If used at the wrong time and by inexperienced hands, a tourniquet can do more harm than good; it may worsen bleeding and cause tissue damage. In an emergency, it can stem severe blood loss from a limb.

A tourniquet is essentially a bandage that, when placed around a limb and tightened, cuts off the blood supply to the part of the limb beyond it. It does this by squeezing closed the arteries (see Arteries and Artery Disease). Its use in medicine goes back thousands of years, but generally a tourniquet is not employed as much today as it was even 50 years ago. A tourniquet has two main purposes. First, in an emergency it can be used to stop major arterial bleeding from a limb.

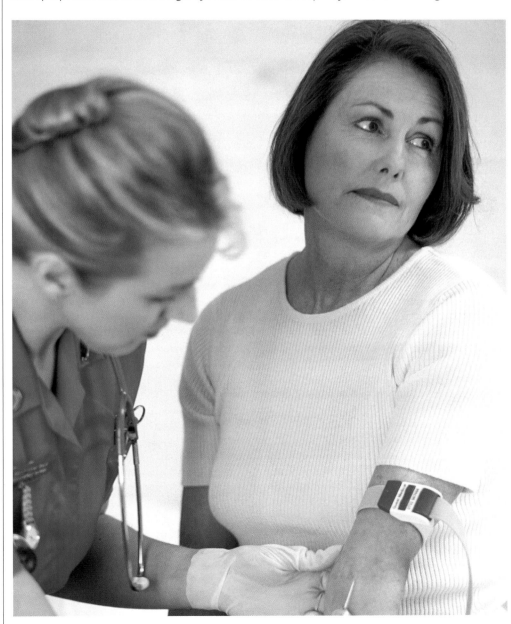

▲ *A venous tourniquet is used to enlarge a vein so that it is a simpler procedure to insert a needle and obtain a blood sample.*

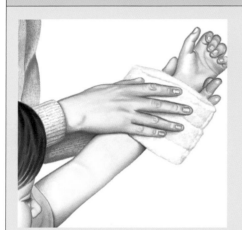

What to do if a limb is bleeding

Get the patient to lie down

Elevate the limb high in the air

Exert direct pressure over the wound, using a handkerchief or a towel as a pad if dressings are not available. Wait for at least five minutes before releasing pressure on the pad and looking underneath to see if bleeding has stopped.

Apply a tourniquet only if the above measures fail to stop pulsed bleeding

Release the tourniquet every 20 minutes

Seek medical help immediately in cases of severe bleeding

Second, it can be used during surgery to provide a blood-free operative area for a surgeon to work on.

The correct application of a tourniquet can, in some circumstances, be lifesaving, but it should be stressed that incorrect use can lead to a worsening of the situation, and even to permanent damage to the limb. Normally it is best to stop bleeding from a limb with firm pressure over the bleeding area and elevation of the limb if the bleeding does not stop.

Dangers

A tourniquet has the potential to be dangerous in several ways. For instance, if it is applied too tightly, or around part of the limb insufficiently covered with muscle, this could lead to damage to the nerves (see Nervous System). Leaving on the tourniquet for too long may cause serious injury, and ultimately tissues can die because they are deprived of blood.

Paradoxically, if the tourniquet is not tight enough, there may be an increase in the amount of bleeding. In this situation if the tourniquet is tight enough to block the veins, where blood is at a very low pressure, but not tight enough to block the arteries, where blood is at high pressure, the blood is still able to get into the limb along the arteries but cannot return through the veins. If there is a cut in a large vein, the bleeding will increase because of the increase in pressure in the veins from blood that is unable to return (see Circulatory System).

Finally, during the period a tourniquet is in place the blood vessels can increase in diameter in response to the lack of oxygenated blood in the limb. On release of the tourniquet these vessels can bleed freely, and actually more heavily than before. Because of all these dangers a tourniquet should not be used to control bleeding unless the person applying it is medically qualified and unless it is absolutely essential.

Use of tourniquets

Before taking the drastic measure of applying a tourniquet, there are certain things that can be tried to stop the bleeding. The first thing to do is to elevate the limb. This causes the blood to be pumped against the force of gravity, and if the bleeding is at the end of the limb it may stop at once. Firm pressure on the bleeding area may

stop the bleeding. In an emergency, a clean handkerchief or a towel will be suitable to use as a pad.

If someone is faced with dealing with bleeding he or she must keep up the pressure for at least five minutes. The use of a tourniquet should be considered only if applying pressure and elevation of the limb fail to stop bleeding or fail to keep the bleeding to a reasonable level. Tourniquets can be made and used in the following way. A bandage, or a handkerchief or scarf, is tied loosely around the limb, over a muscular part, and then tightened by inserting a rod under it, between the limb and the bandage, and twisting the rod so that the bandage tightens. The tourniquet should feel really tight, and there should be an obvious lessening in the amount of bleeding within about half a minute.

If the patient cannot be taken to the hospital immediately, the tourniquet should be released completely every 20 minutes or so to prevent any damage to the limb caused by blood starvation.

Tourniquets in surgery

Tourniquets are also used in planned surgery to enable the surgeon to operate without blood interfering with what he or she is doing. Typically tourniquets are used during surgery on joints, such as cartilage and tendon operations.

The limb is emptied of blood by winding a special rubber bandage tightly around the limb from the end of the limb, toward the body, gradually squeezing out the blood but without losing any. A special tourniquet is then placed around the upper part of the limb. The tourniquet consists of a hollow rubber tube that can be inflated to the desired pressure using a pump. Finally, the rubber bandage is removed and the surgery is then performed.

Other types of tourniquets use compressed gas to apply a controlled amount of pressure to a limb. Some of the systems are computerized and indicate when the time comes to release a tourniquet and also if any problems arise such as malfunctioning equipment or injury to a patient. Modern tourniquet systems consider the size and shape of the limb and also have a limb protection sleeve inside the cuff.

See also: **Blood; Blood pressure; Laboratory tests; Surgery; Veins**

Toxic shock syndrome

Toxic shock syndrome (TSS) was first described in America in 1978, when 90 percent of cases occurred in women who used tampons. Since then, changes in tampon absorbency and composition have led to a decline in cases of TSS.

Toxic shock syndrome (TSS) is a rare but potentially fatal illness. It first became known as a syndrome that affected women who used tampons during their periods, but it is now known that TSS can affect anyone who has any type of Staphylococcus infection, including pneumonia, skin or wound infections, septicemia (blood infection), or osteomyelitis (bone infection). Since TSS was linked to tampon use in 1978, a public health effort resulted in modifications to tampons, which has greatly reduced the number of cases: by 1996, fewer than 100 cases of TSS were reported in the United States, and fewer than half of these were linked to tampon use.

Causes

One of the primary set of conditions that cause TSS seems to be the occurrence of a period, the use of a tampon, and the presence of staphylococci in the vagina. When staphylococci are present

HOW TOXIC SHOCK SYNDROME OCCURS

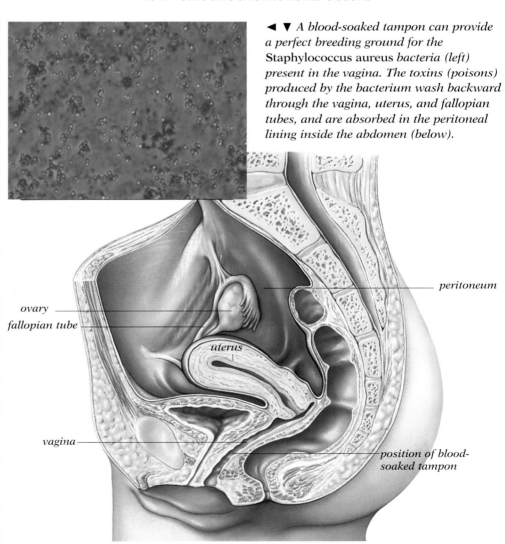

◄ ▼ *A blood-soaked tampon can provide a perfect breeding ground for the* Staphylococcus aureus *bacteria (left) present in the vagina. The toxins (poisons) produced by the bacterium wash backward through the vagina, uterus, and fallopian tubes, and are absorbed in the peritoneal lining inside the abdomen (below).*

ovary

fallopian tube

uterus

vagina

peritoneum

position of blood-soaked tampon

RECOGNIZING THE SYMPTOMS

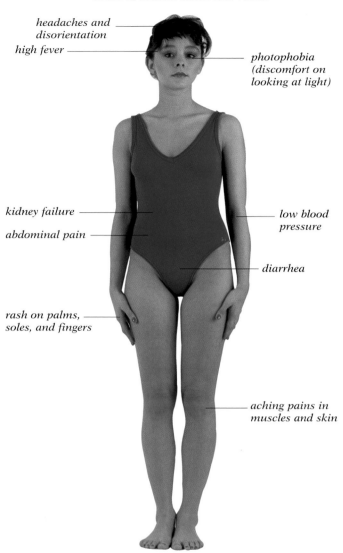

headaches and disorientation

high fever

photophobia (discomfort on looking at light)

kidney failure

abdominal pain

low blood pressure

diarrhea

rash on palms, soles, and fingers

aching pains in muscles and skin

Streptococcal toxic shock syndrome

Strepotococcal toxic shock syndrome (STSS) is a more recent type of toxic shock syndrome, officially recognized only in 1987. SSTS is caused by the entrance of group A Streptococci bacteria into the body—usually through the vagina; skin wounds from cuts, scrapes, or surgery; or chicken pox blisters—that then produce toxins (see Streptococcus). STSS is also a rare syndrome, affecting only about 300 people per year.

Symptoms and dangers

TSS develops suddenly, after an average two-day incubation, with a high fever (over 102.2°F/39°C), headache, dizziness, disorientation, weak and rapid pulse, low blood pressure (shock), rapid breathing, abdominal pain, and vomiting (see Fevers; Shock). Nearly always, painful myalgia resembling flulike symptoms occurs in the muscles and the skin (see Myalgia). During the first 24 hours, watery diarrhea develops in most cases, as well as bloodshot eyes and red under the eyelids or inside the mouth (or the vagina in females). A sunburn-like rash often appears, which may be mistaken for the first flush of fever. Later, it becomes more marked, usually affecting the fingers and sometimes leading to loss of skin from the palms of the hands and the soles of the feet (see Rashes).

As the disease progresses, other problems such as pain in the joints and discomfort on looking toward a light (photophobia) may occur. There will also be failure of at least four of the body's main systems, particularly the liver and kidneys. The kidneys stop passing enough urine to eliminate waste products, so the level of waste products in the blood starts to rise. Kidney failure is probably related to a drop in blood pressure, since the kidneys are sensitive to any changes in the amount of blood flowing to them (see Kidneys and Kidney Diseases). Most patients recover after 10 days, but are left with peeling skin. The death rate is about 5 percent.

STSS shares many of the symptoms of TSS, including low blood pressure, fever, confusion, a weak and rapid pulse, rapid breathing, and liver and kidney failure. There may also be cool, moist, and pale skin; a blotchy rash that may peel; and swollen, red skin surrounding the infected wound. The incubation period for STSS is two to three days.

Treatment and outlook

The most important aspect of the treatment for both TSS and STSS is to quickly replace fluid intravenously to restore the working of the circulation and maintain normal blood pressure. Other problems that can happen have to be faced as they occur; for example, a patient who has difficulty breathing might have to be put on a respirator. In both TSS and STSS, the patient is treated with antibiotics to eradicate the organisms from the body, which can hasten recovery from the illness and prevent the possibility of repeated attacks (see Antibiotics).

Prevention

The main ways for a woman to avoid TSS are to use the lowest absorbency tampon that will handle her menstrual flow, change tampons frequently during a period, wash the hands before and after inserting a tampon, and to remove diaphragms and contraceptive sponges at the correct times. If possible, women should use sanitary pads, rather than tampons, during the later stages of the period. To avoid getting TSS or STSS from skin wounds, people should clean and bandage wounds as soon as possible (see Wounds).

See also: **Sepsis; Staphylococcus**

in the vagina (which they are in many of the cases, but not in all) and a period starts (see Menstruation), the presence of a blood-soaked tampon will provide an excellent culture medium on which the organisms can grow. In most cases, the symptoms result from the production of a toxin (poison) by the staphylococcus, which may then wash backward up through the vagina, uterus, and fallopian tubes to be absorbed by the peritoneal lining inside the abdomen.

The syndrome tends to occur in young women, with an average age of 23; 30 percent of cases involve girls aged between 15 and 21. The risk is greater in younger people because older people are more likely to have the antibodies to protect them from the toxin that causes TSS. The risk of TSS is also greater in women who use high-absorbency tampons. In America, this led to the withdrawal from the market of a tampon made by a certain manufacturer and tighter restrictions on tampon composition and absorbency.

TSS is also more common in women who have left a tampon in place longer than the recommended time, and in women who use diaphragms and contraceptive sponges. It is less common in women who are using a contraceptive pill, perhaps because the amount of menstrual flow is reduced (see Oral Contraceptives).

Trace elements

Questions and Answers

Are trace elements poisonous in excess?

Yes. An example is Wilson's disease, which affects the liver and the brain and results from an excess of copper. Cobalt can be toxic in high doses (20–30 mg a day), and leads to heart failure. Smaller doses can be poisonous if combined with a low-protein diet and a high alcohol intake.

Are extra trace elements essential?

No, a normally balanced diet should contain more than enough of all the trace elements, and it is possible that taking supplements could prove dangerous because many of the trace elements can cause illness if they are present in the body in excessive amounts.

Are trace elements different from the essential minerals in our diet?

No; trace elements are also minerals. They differ from the more important minerals, such as sodium and potassium, only because minute amounts (traces) are required in our diet.

Why are trace elements important?

The bodily functions rely on many chemical reactions continually taking place in a controlled way. The reactions involve the major organic chemical elements carbon, oxygen, and hydrogen. They may also involve other elements in the body, such as sodium or calcium. However, a few of the enzymes that control these interrelated reactions need another substance to work properly. This substance may be a metal, and most of the essential trace elements are metals. An example is zinc, one of the chemical building blocks for vital enzymes, including the enzyme that breaks down alcohol in the liver.

In complex chemical reactions in the human body, trace elements play vital roles. Only minute quantities of trace elements are needed, and an excess, as well as a deficiency, can cause illness.

A balanced diet includes protein, starch, fat, and also the vitamins and minerals that we need to keep us healthy. Because some minerals are required in such tiny amounts, they are called trace elements, since only a tiny amount is required by the body (see Minerals). Most of the requirements of the body are supplied by three elements—carbon, oxygen, and hydrogen—and to a lesser extent nitrogen; kilograms of these substances are taken in every day (see Diet; Nutrition). Relatively large amounts of other elements such as sodium, potassium, and calcium are also required, and a few grams of these elements are found in a normal diet every day. However, trace elements such as copper, selenium, and iodine, which are just as essential for normal life, are needed in only minute quantities. For example, we need only a few milligrams of copper and even less of elements such as iodine and chromium. The body relies on only a few elements to set up the complex and intricate web of chemical reactions essential for health.

What trace elements do

Trace elements have a very important role in bringing about the activity of the various enzymes in the body (see Enzymes). The function of trace elements is to assist in chemical reactions in the body and to act as catalysts. (Although catalysts may initiate a process, they remain unchanged at the end of the reaction.)

All enzymes are proteins, and what each one does depends on the shape into which the long, stringlike protein molecule winds itself. Trace elements play a role because it seems that a few of the body's enzymes require strong chemical forces produced by atoms of certain metallic elements to attain the correct shape for action. Therefore most of the trace elements the body needs are metallic and they either form part of the structure of an enzyme or take part in chemical reactions in the body.

A few trace elements appear to be part of the structure of other important substances in the body. Fluorine is associated with the structure of bones and teeth, and iodine is an essential constituent of the thyroid hormones.

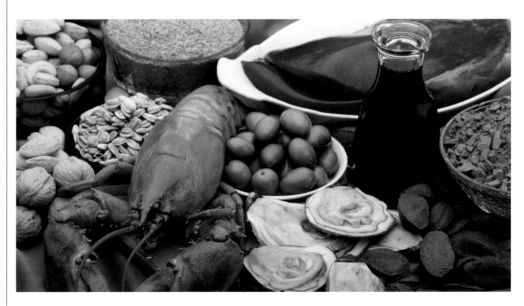

▲ *Lobster, oysters, beef and lamb liver, Brazil nuts, and molasses are rich sources of copper; sunflower seeds, olives, and wheat bran are good sources of copper.*

STRUCTURE OF THYROXINE

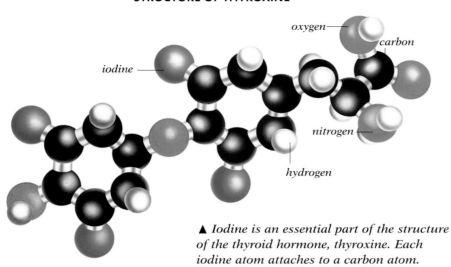

▲ *Iodine is an essential part of the structure of the thyroid hormone, thyroxine. Each iodine atom attaches to a carbon atom.*

Trace elements: Sources and functions

ELEMENT	SOURCE	ROLE
Iron *10 mg	Meat and some green vegetables	Essential for formation of oxygen-carrying pigments hemoglobin (in blood) and myoglobin (in muscle). Deficiency leads to anemia.
Iodine *100 µg	Seafood. Added to salt in US and UK.	Forms part of thyroid hormone. Deficiency results in endemic goiter.
Copper *1.5 mg	Seafood, nuts, vegetable oils	Handles oxygen in cells; helps in formation of blood and melanin. Deficiency may lead to anemia, weakened or impaired respiration and growth, and poor utilization of iron, especially in babies.
Zinc *10–20 mg	Eggs, meat, fish, oats, nuts	Keeps skin healthy. Essential for action of many enzymes. Deficiency leads to retarded growth, late sexual maturation, hair loss, dermatitis, anorexia, vomiting.
Manganese *2–4 mg	Mainly vegetables; also legumes and pasta	Part of several enzymes; essential for activating others. Involved in handling fat and excretion of products of protein breakdown. Deficiency leads to subnormal growth, deficient tissue respiration, menstrual irregularities, trouble in nervous system.
Fluorine *500 µg	Water	Builds healthy teeth and bones. Deficiency contributes to tooth decay and weak bones.
Chromium *10 µg	Water, oils, meat	Deficiency predisposes to diabetes
Selenium *100 µg	Cereals (depends on soil content)	Essential for working of red blood cells. A normal diet ensures there is no deficiency.
Silicon *minute quantity	Vegetables	Forms part of connective tissue structure. A deficiency has no known effect in humans.

*Daily requirement (mg = one-thousandth of a gram; µg = one-millionth of a gram)

Harmful trace elements

Traces of some substances present in food or air are not only of no value but can be positively dangerous. Metals such as lead, mercury, and arsenic are all poisonous in sufficient quantities and have no use in the body. Apart from poisonous metals, it is possible to accumulate high levels of normally beneficial, essential trace elements that then cause illness. In hemochromatosis, an abnormality of the transport of iron in the blood leads to an accumulation of iron in the liver and pancreas. This can cause cirrhosis and diabetes. A genetic-linked disease called Wilson's disease can occur in which the metabolism of copper becomes disorganized, and copper accumulates in the heart and liver.

In other circumstances accidental intake leads to poisoning by metals that are essential in only minute amounts. A notorious example of accidental excess was in Quebec, Canada, where cobalt was added to beer to improve the froth, and therefore put a better head on a glass of beer. This led to an outbreak of heart failure in beer drinkers, as the cobalt slowly poisoned the heart.

Zinc

Zinc is an important trace metal and is found at quite high concentrations in the skin, eyes, liver, pancreas, and bone.

An important discovery about zinc was the realization that deficiency leads to disease. In some parts of Egypt and Iran there is a deficiency of zinc in the diet; here, there is a tendency for boys not to mature properly, and not to go through puberty. Adding zinc to the diet of these boys brings about rapid maturation (see Puberty).

More relevant is the role that zinc plays in healing the skin. Zinc given in tablet form can speed up healing of various wounds. In recent years, a disease called acrodermatitis enteropathica has been recognized, in which the skin produces eczemalike symptoms, particularly in infants being weaned. The condition results from poor absorption of zinc, and it responds well to zinc treatment.

See also: Skin and skin diseases

Tracheostomy

Questions and Answers

Is it possible to speak with a tracheostomy, and does it have long-term effects on the voice?

Usually, it is not possible to speak with a tracheostomy in the first few weeks. However, a special tube can be inserted after a while, and covering the outside end of the tube with a finger lets air go up into the larynx. The voice may be weaker after a tracheotomy, but should eventually regain its normal strength, depending, of course, on the original reason for surgery.

Is it easy to do an emergency tracheotomy if someone is choking to death?

No. A tracheotomy may seem simple, but it is not. However, if you are sure that the obstruction is at the back of the throat and if all else has failed—that is, the obstruction cannot be removed through the mouth or by performing the Heimlich maneuver, and there is no chance of finding a medical person—a cricothyroidotomy is an easier procedure. A small cut is made about 1 in. (2.5 cm) below the Adam's apple until the windpipe is entered.

If someone has a temporary tracheostomy, is it necessary to have another operation to close the opening in the neck?

No, not always. Usually, as soon as the tracheostomy tube is taken out the hole starts getting smaller. Eventually, it should heal up on its own, but if there is a persistent leak, minor surgery may be done.

For how long can someone have a tracheostomy?

If it is temporary, an effort will be made to remove it, but many people have had one for years.

Blockage of the windpipe from disease or injury, or paralysis of breathing, can be rapidly fatal. In such cases, a tracheotomy—surgically creating an opening in the trachea—can be a lifesaver.

The word "tracheotomy" comes from two Greek words: *trachea*, the windpipe; and *tomy*, to cut. It should not be confused with the word "tracheostomy," which is derived from *stoma* (a mouth), and is the actual opening in the trachea. Tracheotomy means the surgical act of making that opening.

When is it necessary?

There are various reasons for performing a tracheotomy. Sometimes it is performed because of an obstruction in the upper part of the windpipe. Making an opening below the obstruction will allow the patient to breathe until the obstruction can be removed. The obstruction can be a result of injury to the mouth or the back of the throat; inflammation (see Inflammation), causing swelling of the upper airway; or a tumor in the larynx (see Larynx and Laryngitis). It may be sudden or gradual in onset, and consequently the tracheotomy may have to be performed as emergency surgery or as planned surgery.

Sometimes the tracheotomy forms part of another surgical procedure. For instance, a tumor of the larynx (voice box) may sometimes necessitate the removal of the larynx. After this procedure the patient will have a permanent tracheostomy.

CREATING A TRACHEOSTOMY

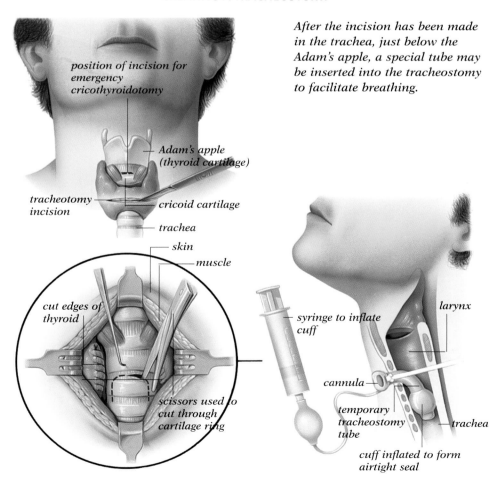

After the incision has been made in the trachea, just below the Adam's apple, a special tube may be inserted into the tracheostomy to facilitate breathing.

position of incision for emergency cricothyroidotomy

Adam's apple (thyroid cartilage)

tracheotomy incision

cricoid cartilage

trachea

skin

muscle

cut edges of thyroid

scissors used to cut through cartilage ring

syringe to inflate cuff

larynx

cannula

temporary tracheostomy tube

trachea

cuff inflated to form airtight seal

A tracheotomy may be performed when a patient has to be attached to a respirator for a long period of time. This will usually be performed as a planned procedure and is most commonly done because the person has lost the ability to breathe naturally, for example, as a result of paralysis caused by disease or following an accident. A patient who has lost the ability to keep saliva and other secretions out of the trachea because of coma or a specific swallowing problem may also require a tracheotomy.

For short periods, a tube can be passed through the mouth or nose into the trachea, but if these tubes are left in place for more than about seven to 10 days, the lining of the trachea may become damaged. This could lead later on to narrowing of the trachea. Another advantage of performing a tracheotomy in this situation is that the dead space—the space that is taken up by the air in the mouth and the air passages—is greatly diminished, making breathing more efficient. Also, sucking out unwanted secretions from the chest in a patient who cannot cough is much easier when the suction tube can be passed through the tracheostomy and straight down into the lungs.

How it is done

A tracheotomy may be performed under local or general anesthesia. The surgeon first makes an incision in the patient's skin overlying the trachea, in the midline halfway between the Adam's apple and the top end of the sternum (breastbone). The tissues under the skin are divided, and the trachea is exposed. Quite often there is a band of tissue across the front of the trachea. This is part of the thyroid gland (see Thyroid), and it has to be divided between ligatures or it will bleed profusely. A small vertical incision is then made in the trachea itself and a metal or plastic tube is inserted. If the patient cannot breathe unaided, the tube is connected to a respirator.

After surgery, the hole between the trachea and the skin of the neck, which is called the tracheostomy, has to be kept open using one of these special tubes. If the tube were not left in the trachea, the opening would gradually close; in fact, if a tracheostomy is to be only temporary, then it will eventually be allowed to close when it is no longer needed by simply taking out the tube and waiting for the hole to close on its own.

A week or so after the tracheotomy has been performed, the tube will be taken out for a few minutes, and then it will be reinserted. Later, when the tissues have formed a definite track, the patient can change his or her own tube.

Problems with tracheostomies

There are a number of complications associated with tracheostomies, such as blockage of the tube, hemorrhage from veins around the trachea, and narrowing of the trachea. However, the main problem from a patient's point of view is that he or she cannot speak. Air is diverted away from the larynx, and so cannot make the vocal cords sound (see Speech; Vocal Cords). This can sometimes be overcome later on by the insertion of a special tracheostomy tube that has a valve in it to allow air to pass out of the lungs up into the larynx, provided that the patient covers up the outlet with his or her finger.

A tracheotomy is rarely used in emergency situations, for example when a person is choking. Apart from the obvious disadvantages of doing anything that would take time in a critical situation, it would be very difficult to assess the location of the

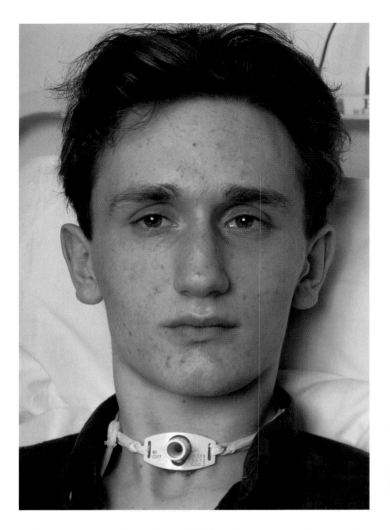

▲ *A tracheotomy is performed if the windpipe is obstructed because of injury, or a blockage of some kind, or a disease. Usually the tracheostomy will be only temporary.*

obstruction. If the trachea was obstructed below the point where a tracheotomy is usually performed, then there would be no reason to do it. The obstruction has to be sited at the back of the mouth or throat, or in the larynx, for a tracheotomy to be effective.

If a person is choking on, say, a piece of food during a meal, someone should immediately try to remove the foreign body that is causing the obstruction. This might be possible by passing a finger into the mouth and trying to hook the object out, or by performing the Heimlich maneuver.

Cricothyroidotomy

In an emergency, an operation called a cricothyroidotomy may be performed. This involves cutting a hole in the lower part of the larynx, where it joins the trachea between the thyroid and cricoid cartilages. The advantage of a cricothyroidotomy over a tracheotomy is that this part of the windpipe is nearer to the surface of the skin, so surgery can be performed much more quickly. The disadvantage is that it may cause permanent weakness of the voice, and possibly also permanent narrowing of the air passages.

> See also: **Surgery; Tumors**

Traction

Traction may appear to be a crude and rather old-fashioned form of treatment, but it is as yet unsurpassed as a valuable way of dealing with many painful conditions of the skeleton, including fractures and dislocations.

How long does traction last before taking effect?

This depends on the condition it is being used to treat. In the case of a fractured thighbone (femur), it has to last until the bone is strong enough for normal movement and weight bearing—anything up to three to four months. If the traction is removed too soon, the bone may refracture or slowly bend through the healing fracture to cause a deformity. However, the time can be reduced by combining traction with other treatments. When traction is used to treat a dislocated hip, the joint needs to be rested for several weeks to prevent further damage. When traction is used to relieve back and neck pain, it can be applied either for short periods once or twice a day, or for continuous periods of one to two weeks.

Is traction more effective in children because their bones are still growing?

Traction does not cause a bone to grow faster. For example, you couldn't make a short leg longer in a child simply by applying traction to it for a long time. Traction is often used in children for fractures of the thighbone or femur, as a safe, effective way of getting the fracture to heal in a good position.

Can you have a course of traction as an outpatient?

Yes. This is called intermittent traction. It is used for many types of back pain, such as a slipped disk. It is usually done in the physical therapy department, and combined with other treatments such as heat and exercise. Traction relieves painful muscle spasms by pulling gently in the opposite direction. Sometimes it also pulls the vertebrae slightly so that the slipped disk moves away from the crushed nerve, lessening the pain.

The most common use of traction is in dealing with types of fracture. The purpose is to stop the fracture from moving, and thereby causing pain, and to pull the bone along its length to prevent it from shortening. The fractures most often treated in this way are those of the thighbone, or femur. Such fractures are unsuitable for treating in plaster, since to immobilize the femur it would be necessary to apply a bulky and uncomfortable cast, including part of the body and the whole leg. Traction may also be used in fractures of the shinbone (tibia), pelvis, spine, and elbow.

Certain dislocations, particularly those of the hip, may also be treated with traction (see Dislocation). This is the safest way of resting the stretched and torn tissues, and of preventing further damage. Traction may also be used to relieve painful conditions of the back and the neck, such as the extremely common slipped disk, and to overcome joint deformities.

How traction works

When a bone or joint becomes painful, through injury or disease, the surrounding muscles contract in an effort to stabilize and protect the painful part. This prolonged contraction is called muscle spasm, and it is a reflex action that the individual cannot control (see Reflexes). This may be painful in itself, and may be more painful than the underlying condition. Since not all the muscles in the body are equally powerful, the pull of the contracting muscles may cause a deformity in the limb. The main function of traction is to overcome this painful muscle spasm by pulling steadily and firmly in the opposite direction from the contracting muscles. At the same time, the physical deformity is improved or eliminated. In the case of a fracture, the bones are not actually pulled apart, since the intact muscles, ligaments, and tendons prevent overstretching.

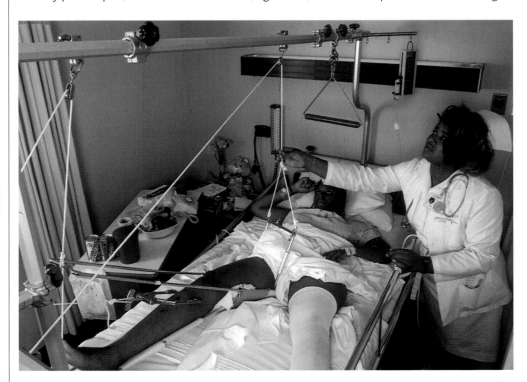

▲ *The complicated modern apparatus belies the simplicity of the principle—only one cord and weight actually perform the traction on the limb.*

Do you always need physical therapy after traction?

No; this depends entirely on the condition for which traction is being applied. It is often used for major fractures and dislocations, and when it is stopped, physical therapy may be needed to help strengthen muscles and to get stiff joints moving. However, when there are no such problems the patient could simply exercise by returning to normal activities.

Do hospitals have special floors for people in traction?

Patients in traction need a lot of nursing care. The traction apparatus must be watched and adjusted frequently, areas of pressure relieved, and the patients' ordinary needs tended. This is done by a team of nurses, doctors, orthopedic technicians, and physical therapists. Larger hospitals often have an orthopedic floor where patients in traction are cared for, but this can also be done on general floors.

Why doesn't putting traction on a broken leg pull the fracture apart?

In a fracture the bone is broken but the other tissues are largely intact. The pull of the traction is enough to keep the fractured bones at the right length for healing, and this is checked by taking X rays. It is surprisingly difficult to pull the fractured ends apart too much, because of the strength of the soft tissues—the muscles, ligaments, and tendons.

Is it possible to move about while in traction?

Yes, a lot of movement is possible in most forms of traction. The weights are suspended by pulleys arranged so that the direction of the pull is the same whether the patient is sitting or lying. Also, the limb joints can be moved without disturbing the pull, and the joints and muscles can be exercised while the fracture is healing.

SKIN TRACTION

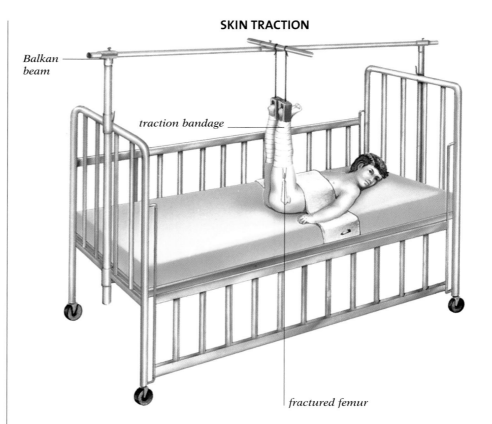

Balkan beam

traction bandage

fractured femur

▲ *Skin traction involves applying force indirectly to the bone or joint by means of weights and an adhesive bandage.*

The technique

In order to apply a firm and steady pull along the length of a limb, some form of weight is needed, and also some means of attaching it to the patient. This can be done either by attaching the weight directly to the skeleton—skeletal traction—or indirectly by sticking it to the skin (see Skeleton). Skeletal traction is applied by putting a metal pin through the appropriate bone then attaching the necessary weights to the pin.

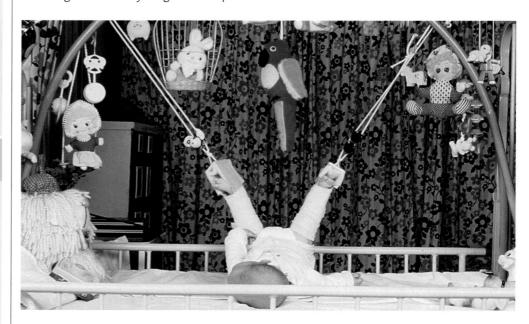

▲ *Traction, using pulleys, is used to treat a baby born with congenital hip dislocation.*

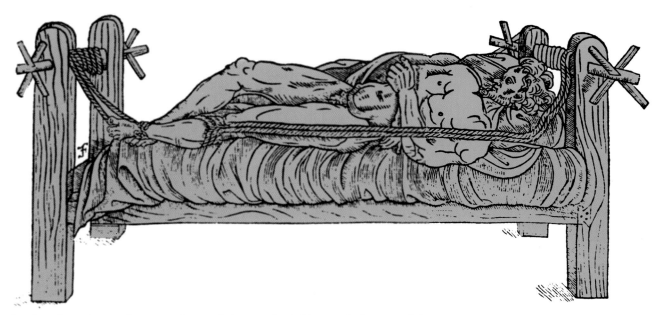

▲ *Traction has been in use for centuries, so it has undeniably stood the test of time.*

Skin traction is applied by means of adhesive tape that is applied to a large area of skin on the limb. The traction force is indirectly applied to the bone or joint, just as when a person pulls on his or her finger, and it pulls on the underlying bone. The disadvantage of this method is that if too much weight is applied, the adhesive tape slides or pulls off—so it cannot be used when more than about 8 pounds (3.6 kg) of traction is needed.

The weights are attached to the traction pin, or tape, by cords that run over pulleys at the foot of the bed. With fractures, the limb is often rested on a splint to give further support and comfort, and other weights and pulleys may be used to suspend the splint.

The pulleys are hung from a metal frame above the bed called a Balkan beam. This is why traction often looks very complicated, but usually only one cord and weight are actually performing the traction. Once the apparatus is established, the pull of the weights tends to draw the patient toward the end of the bed, a problem that can be overcome by elevating the foot of the bed slightly.

Another traction method is to use the patient's own weight; this is often done with children up to age two who have fractures of the femur. Both legs have skin traction bandages applied and they are tied to a beam directly overhead, with the buttocks suspended just off the bed. Thus the child's own weight provides the traction force.

Spinal problems require slightly different techniques. Simple spinal traction may be applied by means of a girdle that is placed around the pelvis or, when the neck is involved, by a halter that fits closely around the chin and the back of the neck. For those spinal injuries in which a stronger and more prolonged pull is needed, skeletal traction may be applied by means of skull tongs. The sharp ends of the tongs are actually embedded in the outer bone of the skull just above the ears, and strong traction can then be applied to the neck.

How long does it last?

Traction may be the only form of treatment used in a fracture, in which case it must be maintained until the bone is strong enough for ordinary walking, sitting, and turning. In the case of a fractured femur this may be up to three or four months.

Time spent in traction can be reduced by combining it with other forms of treatment. A fractured femur may be in traction until it is more stable, and then a type of walking cast can be applied to the limb so that the patient can start to walk with the help of crutches. Other fractures are treated with only a week or two in traction to allow the early acute swelling and any skin injuries to settle. A cast is then applied or surgery performed.

A patient with a slipped disk may have one or two weeks of continuous traction, or the traction may be applied for 30 minutes to an hour each day in conjunction with physical therapy. This can, of course, be done as outpatient treatment for several weeks if necessary (see Outpatients; Physical Therapy).

Advantages and disadvantages

Traction has been used in roughly its present form since the early 19th century, so it is a tried and tested method. One advantage is that because no external splinting or bandaging is needed, an injured limb can be watched carefully for any sign of complications. Also, because the joints are left free, early movement after an injury is possible, preventing stiffness and maintaining muscle strength. In severe injuries of the bone, the length and general alignment of the limb can be maintained while the patient is awaiting any further treatment.

However, there are disadvantages, too. Although the traction pins give little trouble, and most patients are comfortable once they have settled into the traction apparatus, lying in bed for a long period can create complications. A young patient can withstand weeks in bed without any serious problems, other than boredom. However, the physical effects of prolonged rest in bed are more severe in the elderly. These effects include pressure sores (see Bedsores), muscle weakening, softening of the bones, pneumonia, urinary infections, and thrombosis. Such risks have led surgeons to treat fractures in the elderly by other means, such as by surgery, so that the person can get up and walk as soon as possible.

See also: **Back and backache; Fractures; Joints; Slipped disk**

Tranquilizers

Although most people seek peace and tranquillity, feelings of tension and anxiety can be experienced for a variety of reasons. Tranquilizers are sometimes prescribed to restore calmness and to help people cope.

Everyone can cope with some stress in his or her life, and some people even thrive on it. However, there are times when people feel particularly anxious for a definite reason, and other times when there is no clear or obvious reason for their anxiety. Medical science has developed a variety of drugs to treat stress and anxiety; their general name is tranquilizers or anxiolytic drugs, but some of these drugs are called sedatives (see Anxiety; Stress).

Major tranquilizers
Many different types of drugs are used as tranquilizers and their actions and uses are also different. The main division is into major and minor tranquilizers. The major tranquilizers are used for the treatment of psychotic states, in which the working of the mind is disturbed. They are of help in treating some of the major mental disorders such as schizophrenia, hallucinations, and mania (hence their name), as well as a number of other conditions including anxiety. Among the best-known major tranquilizers are chlorpromazine (Largactil) and trifluoperazine (Stelazine). Most are taken by mouth, but some can be given by "depot" injections. This is the term for an injection of a chemical that is actually stored in the body and remains effective for weeks.

An important advantage of the major tranquilizers is that they do not produce dependence. Their principal side effect is muscle stiffness and shakiness, but this stops when the drug is discontinued. Muscle stiffness can also affect the face and mouth, or the eye muscles; this stiffness can be distressing if the patient does not know the cause. Often another drug is prescribed to control these unwanted effects (see Side Effects).

Minor tranquilizers
The minor tranquilizers have a depressant effect on the brain and slow down its working. There are three principal types of drug in this group: the benzodiazepines, the beta-blockers, and the drug buspirone. Barbiturates are no longer used. The benzodiazepines are used as antianxiety

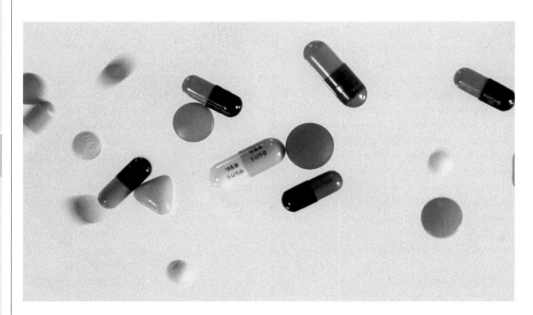

▲ *One of these highly effective tranquilizers can relieve anything from psychoses to insomnia and stress.*

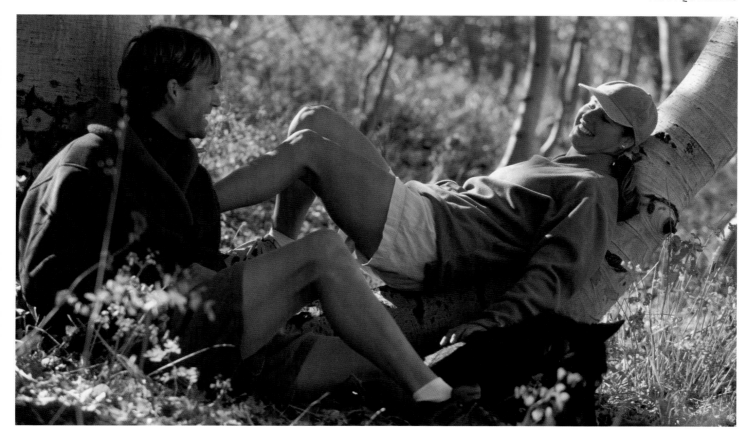

▲ *When stress occurs it is tempting to take a pill to control it, but getting away from it all may bring the relief we need.*

drugs, as sleeping pills, and also to control epilepsy. In small doses they act as tranquilizers, and a larger dose produces sleep.

Benzodiazepine is the family name for such well-known drugs as diazepam (Valium), nitrazepam (Mogadon), and chlordiazepoxide (Librium). These are the drugs that most people refer to when tranquilizers are mentioned. They have been in use for about 20 years, and are the most widely used drugs in the world.

They are generally given in relatively small doses during the day, and have a sedative or calming effect on the mind. This is the main reason why they are effective at relieving anxiety and tension. If the dose is too high, they will cause drowsiness or sleepiness. But this is part of their sedative effect, and if they are given in sufficiently high doses they produce sleep. Their main uses are as antianxiety drugs, and as sleeping pills, and their record for safety is remarkable. Taken in overdose, they can produce profound sleep or coma, but fatal overdoses are rare. Addiction is known but is uncommon. Someone taking them regularly who then suddenly stops may have a few nights of disturbed sleep or nightmares, but serious withdrawal symptoms are actually rare (see Withdrawal Symptoms).

Tranquilizers should be used only as a short-term remedy. When someone is troubled by real anxiety or stress, a course of tranquilizers for a week or two may be very helpful in restoring his or her equanimity. Similarly, if a person is unable to sleep these drugs may help to reestablish a normal sleep pattern.

However, it is being increasingly recognized that these drugs are of very little use when given for long periods, since their effectiveness rapidly falls off.

Beta-blocking drugs

When a person is really anxious several things happen in the body as a result of overactivity of the sympathetic nervous system (see Autonomic Nervous System). The muscles are tense and may even tremble. The heart beats rapidly, the hands become sweaty, the mouth becomes dry, and there is a feeling of butterflies in the stomach. All these feelings can develop from acute stress, such as speaking or playing a musical instrument in front of a large audience, or taking examinations. If the stress is prolonged, the symptoms may sometimes be equally prolonged. A person with a highly anxious personality may focus on the symptoms that are produced by anxiety; for example, he or she may worry about sweating hands (see Tension).

Beta-blockers are a group of drugs that block the actions of the sympathetic nervous system, and are widely used in treating high blood pressure and heart disorders. However, they can also help someone faced with an acutely stressful situation, such as performing in public, to do the job without the distraction of the symptoms from his or her own body. They can also sometimes help to break up the symptoms of chronic anxiety, but they do not have the calming effect that tranquilizers have on the mind. Doctors quite often prescribe low doses of beta-blocking drugs for people who are troubled by anxiety symptoms or who go to pieces under stress (see Symptoms).

Buspirone

Buspirone has the brand name BuSpar, and it is quite different, both chemically and in its pharmacological action, from the benzodiazepines. It is not a muscle relaxant and it has no value in controlling seizures. The mode of its action as a tranquilizer is obscure although it is known to be capable of blocking serotonin

Prozac: the happiness drug?

Fluoxetine is the generic name for a drug that has aroused more public interest than almost any other. Sometimes known as the "happiness pill," this drug —best known under the name Prozac—has now been prescribed to over 40 million people worldwide. Many doctors and users claim it is capable of entirely altering a patient's mood and outlook, from pessimism to optimism, removing sensitivity to criticism, and totally altering his or her state of mind for the better.

Prozac is one of a group of drugs called the selective serotonin reuptake inhibitors (SSRIs). Serotonin, or 5-HT, is a natural chemical substance that stimulates nerves and hence brain activity, and low amounts of it are thought to cause depression. Normally serotonin is pulled back into the nerve ending that releases it, but Prozac and its sister drugs prevent this, so that serotonin is able to act for a longer period, causing greater nerve stimulation.

Prozac is an effective mood enhancer, and has comparatively minor obvious side effects. It does not, for example, effect noradrenaline levels and does not cause drowsiness—a criticism often aimed at other antidepressant drugs. Moreover, because it remains in the body a long time, only one capsule needs to be taken daily (usually in the morning).

The drug can, however, cause loss of both appetite, weight, and libido, sexual dysfunction, nausea, anxiety, skin rashes, itching, insomnia, and tremors. Perhaps a more subtle effect is that people who use it need no longer make the effort to organize their lives in a way that brings them contentment and satisfaction. Reports throughout the 1990s suggested that Prozac had caused suicidal thoughts in patients and some deaths, but lawsuits against the drug's manufacturers Eli Lilly and Company, Inc. have generally been unsuccessful; the drug has not been scientifically proven to cause such reactions.

Prozac is used primarily to treat depression, obsessive-compulsive disorder, bulimia nervosa, and severe symptoms of premenstrual syndrome. Most doctors will prescribe Prozac only to patients who are genuinely ill, but there is a small but vocal school of thought that believes that the drug is justified for anyone who thinks that life is not as pleasant as it ought to be. One practitioner was said, at one stage, to have prescribed Prozac or other reuptake inhibitors to every one of his patients. Perhaps significantly, this practitioner was investigated by the State Board of Psychology.

There are some firm guidelines when using Prozac. Anyone who is considering using the drug should tell their doctor about any liver, kidney, or heart problems they may have.
The safety of using the drug during pregnancy or breast-feeding is not entirely established, so be sure to discuss these issues with your doctor.
People over the age of 60 are more likely to suffer from adverse side effects, and it it likely, therefore, that a doctor will prescribe a reduced dose.

When taking Prozac, avoid drinking alcohol, as this can greatly increase the sedative effects of the drug, and don't drive or engage in hazardous work until you are sure of how drowsy the drug is going to make you feel.

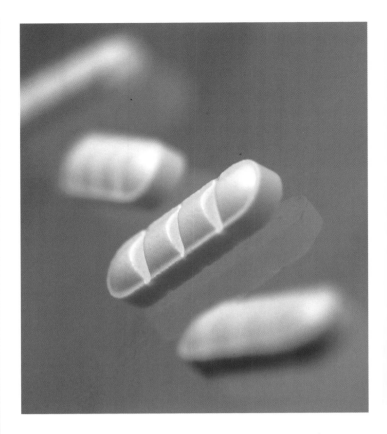

▲ *Benzodiazepines are commonly used antianxiety drugs, also known as tranquilizers.*

receptors on nerve cells. It has a less powerful sedative effect than the benzodiazepines and is less likely to produce addiction. It does not appear to interact with alcohol or with other depressants of the nervous system. It is effective in relieving the symptoms of anxiety within one to three weeks, whether or not these are associated with depression. However, it is licensed for short-term use only. Side effects are uncommon but may include excitement, light-headedness, and nausea.

Alternatives to tranquilizers

For any sudden or severe mental stress, many people recommend a cup of tea or coffee, a cigarette, or an alcoholic drink. Tea, coffee, and cigarettes may not relieve tension or anxiety, but being cared for and using the hands can be reassuring. Alcohol, on the other hand, has a definite sedative effect, and may be useful in a stressful situation, but it should not be relied on regularly as a tranquilizer. People who use alcohol in this way should seek medical advice before the situation gets out of hand.

Alternatives to tranquilizers vary from herbal remedies to jogging and yoga. However, perhaps the most important antidote is to see problems in perspective and to look for solutions rather than difficulties. Keeping lines of communication open is important, and a frank discussion may relieve tension. If people can adapt and change their way of life and attitude, most of them should be able to cope with stress, and will rarely need drugs to control anxiety.

See also: Alcoholism;
Injections; Stress management

Transdermal patch

Transdermal patches are a comparatively recent and valuable addition to the ways in which medication can be administered. The range of drugs that can be delivered in this way has been growing steadily.

Transdermal (through the skin) drug delivery systems have been in use to a very limited extent for many years, but it is only recently that techniques have been developed that have allowed a considerable extension of the method. Because of the relatively thick and waterproof epidermis, the skin is normally impermeable to many substances, but there are various solvents that will increase the permeability of the skin to allow a passage through it into the blood vessels below the skin. Transdermal patches are layered devices consisting of an absorbent layer of the

Questions and Answers

Delivering drugs by skin patches seems to be widespread. When did the practice start?

The first transdermal patch was introduced in 1981, but to begin with, progress was slow. When it became apparent that HRT could be provided in this way, the popularity of the system rapidly increased. For a time HRT dominated the skin patch scene, but in recent years the range of medication that can effectively be given in this way has widened.

Is there any real advantage in taking drugs by skin patch rather than by mouth, or is it just a gimmick to improve the profits of the drug manufacturers?

Transdermal drug delivery offers some real advantages. It allows drugs to be passed into the bloodstream at a steady and relatively uniform dose rate. It solves the problem of drugs that upset the stomach. Administration of a drug can be stopped at any time by removing the patch. Perhaps the greatest advantage, however, is that a continuous, even supply of the drug can be given over a period of days. This can be much more effective than taking a tablet three times a day.

Which drugs can be taken by skin patch?

For postmenopausal women, estradiol, an estrogen, is used to prevent estrogen-deficiency effects and the drug alendronate to combat osteoporosis. Progestin and estrogen are used in patch form as a contraceptive. Glyceryl trinitrate is used to control angina pectoris, and testosterone patches relieve male sex-hormone deficiency. Clonidine patches treat high blood pressure; nicotine patches are used as an aid to quit smoking. Fentanyl patches control severe, prolonged pain.

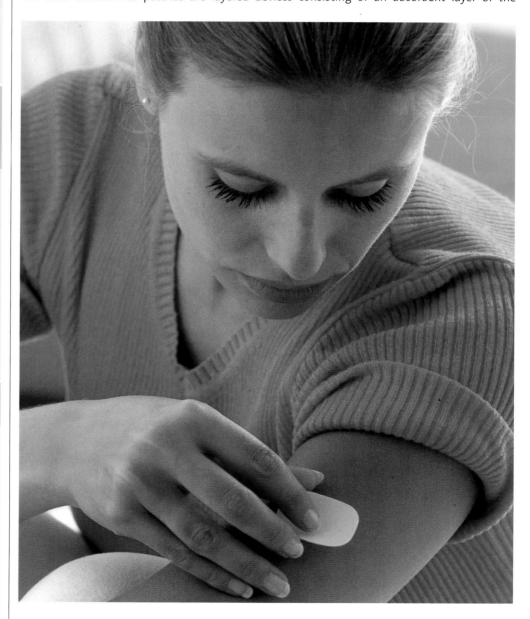

▲ *A woman applies a nicotine patch to her arm in an effort to quit smoking. The patch delivers a measured dose of nicotine to beat the craving for a cigarette.*

permeating solution, a layer of the drug, and a controlling membrane through which the drug diffuses to reach the skin. The patches must be applied to non-hairy skin and should not be applied repeatedly to exactly the same skin site.

Advantages

Drugs taken by mouth undergo a delay in absorption and then pass into the bloodstream. All of the drug acquired in this way then passes directly to the liver, where up to 90 percent of it may be altered and rendered useless. This effect is termed "first-pass metabolism" and its result is that the effective dose of a drug is greatly reduced. First-pass metabolism is avoided when drugs are given by skin patch. Once a drug is distributed in the circulation and in body fluids the rate of breakdown by the liver is much reduced. Patches also bypass the stomach and intestines.

Disadvantages

However, only a small number of drugs are currently suitable for delivery by a transdermal route. This number is likely to increase with further research. A major limitation of the method is that the greater the size of the drug molecules, the less easily they will pass through the skin. Many people develop local allergic reactions to adhesive patches. There are also considerable differences in the rate of diffusion through the skin of different people, so dosage may have to be adjusted. Another unexpected disadvantage has come to light in recent years. Not only can patches come adrift; they can become accidentally stuck to the wrong person. There are an increasing number of reports that the partners of patients suffer unexpected, and for a time inexplicable, symptoms as a result of this effect. Even small children who have been taken into bed for comforting have been affected in this way.

Commonly used patches

HRT estradiol skin patches such as Estraderm are available in strengths of 25, 50, 75, and 100 micrograms. These must be replaced every three or four days and applied to a different area of the skin. The administration of HRT is now questioned, owing to adverse research reports that show that there may be an increase in heart disease and breast cancer in certain women taking HRT.

Progestin and estrogen: A birth control patch for women called Ortho Evra was approved by the Food and Drug Administration (FDA) in 2001. The patch delivers two synthetic hormones—progestin (norelgestromin) and estrogen (ethinyl estradiol)—which prevent ovulation and thus pregnancy. It is applied to the skin of the abdomen, upper torso, upper outer arm, or buttocks on the day after the woman's period ends. After one week, it is replaced with a new patch to one of the other mentioned sites. This is repeated each week until the fourth week, when no patch is applied and the menstrual period occurs. When used correctly, it is 99 percent effective.

Nitroglycerine: Transderm Nitro is an example of a skin patch that delivers nitroglycerine for the prevention of the pain of angina pectoris. Patches contain either 5 or 10 milligrams of the drug and may be used continuously or intermittently. A new patch must be applied every 24 hours. These patches can be used to prevent vein inflammation (phlebitis) following the use of cannulas that have to be left in veins for two days or longer.

Nicotine: Nicotine transdermal patches are available in strengths that provide 5 mg, 10 mg, or 15 mg, over the course of 16 hours.

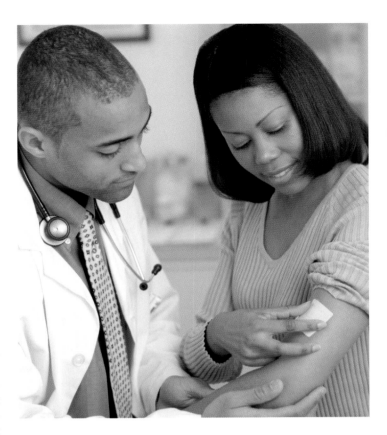

▲ *A drug available in a patch is administered by a doctor.*

The usual course is to apply the 15-mg patch once a day for 8 weeks, then the 10-mg patch daily for 2 weeks and, finally, the 5-mg daily for 2 weeks (see Nicotine).

Testosterone: Transdermal patches of testosterone are available that deliver either 2.5 mg or 5 mg of the hormone over 24 hours. A new patch is applied before the patient goes to bed each night.

Fentanyl: Durogesic is a skin patch containing the powerful opioid painkiller Fentanyl. It is used especially to control severe and persistent pain in cancer and other diseases. Self-adhesive Fentanyl skin patches come in four different strengths—25, 50, 75, and 100 micrograms—and these patches deliver this microgram dosage of the drug every hour for a period of 72 hours. Dosage is controlled by starting with the lowest-dosage patch and then, if necessary, moving on to patches of higher dosage.

The future

The future seems bright for transdermal delivery of drugs, and considerable research is in progress. A principal difficulty is the question of the molecular size of many drugs. Drugs like insulin are proteins and pass through the skin with great difficulty. It would be a boon to diabetics if their insulin could be taken in this simple, painless, and nondamaging way rather than by repeated daily injections. Insulin cannot be taken by mouth, because it would be digested and destroyed in the intestine, but if it can be delivered to the bloodstream through the skin from a patch the effect would be the same as that of an injection. Many problems remain to be solved, however.

> *See also:* **Diabetes; Pain; Pain management; Smoking**

Transient ischemic attack

Questions and Answers

Every person over the age of 40 should know what a transient ischemic attack (TIA) is, what it signifies, and how it is caused. This knowledge could be important enough to be lifesaving.

I am worried about my mother. She keeps complaining that she can't see anything to her right side, then, after half an hour or so, she says that her vision is back to normal. Should she have her eyes tested? What could be causing this?

You are right to be worried. Your mother's problem has nothing to do with her eyes. She is suffering from periods of what is called homonymous hemianopia. This can't be caused by the eyes and is always an indication of a defect of brain function. Your mother is having transient ischemic attacks affecting the visual part of her brain and urgently needs to see a physician, preferably a neurologist.

My girlfriend is 17. She tells me that she often has a small area of blindness in both eyes that expands slowly and has a sparkling edge. This occurs over a period of about 20 minutes and then clears up. I have been looking this up and it sounds to me like a transient ischemic attack. Should she see a doctor?

Although she may never have a severe headache, your friend is having attacks of a form of migraine. It might be a good idea for her to have a medical checkup, but you can be sure she is not having transient ischemic attacks. Both her age and the description of the symptom are against it.

If a person is having a transient ischemic attack that passes off, is the brain actually being damaged?

It's possible to be sure about this only if the attack is followed by residual loss of function. If it is, then the brain has certainly been damaged. However, even if there are no indications of functional loss, some damage may have been caused that could be cumulative if other attacks occur.

"Ischemia" means a local inadequacy in blood supply. Transient ischemic attacks (TIAs) are brief episodes of disturbance of the body's function resulting from malfunction of part of the brain because the blood supply to that part of the brain is temporarily interrupted or reduced. TIAs are more common in men than in women and in most cases imply that a fairly severe level of the artery disease atherosclerosis is present (see Arteries and Artery Disease).

TIAs are important warning signs of impending stroke and must never be ignored. About a quarter of the people who suffer a TIA will have a fatal or nonfatal stroke within five years. Many of them will have a stroke or a heart attack within a year. Although a heart attack has nothing to do with the brain, the reason is that the same arterial disease, atherosclerosis, that causes TIAs and strokes also causes blockage of the coronary arteries of the heart (see Coronary Arteries and Thrombosis; Heart Attack).

Definition and types

TIAs have, for many years, been defined as disturbances of function lasting for less than 24 hours. This arbitrary definition is now being challenged by the view that it is important to distinguish between isolated attacks that last for a few minutes or even up to one hour, and those of longer

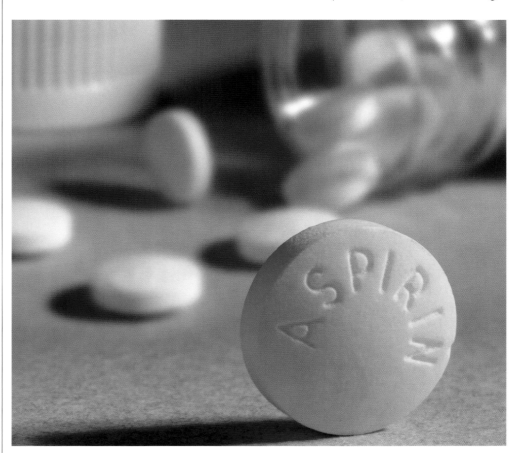

▲ *A small daily dose of aspirin is a recommended treatment to people who have suffered TIAs because it helps to prevent blood clots that can lead to a stroke.*

duration. It is also now believed important to distinguish between a single brief episode that passes quickly, and repeated episodes of the same kind.

Symptoms

TIAs may take many forms—a period of obscuration of vision, brief weakness or paralysis in an arm or leg, weakness down one side of the body, local numbness, speech difficulty, loss of the ability to name objects, loss of part of the field of vision, and so on (see Paralysis). Because doctors now know accurately the location of all the major functions of the brain, they can tell from the type of disturbance which area of the brain is affected (see Brain). It is usually possible to tell which arteries are involved.

Most TIAs last for two to 15 minutes. The first one experienced may be followed shortly by a stroke of any degree of severity. Or a stroke may occur only after many TIAs have occurred over a period of weeks, months, or even years. It even happens sometimes that a person may have TIAs which then cease, leaving no discernable permanent paralysis. This is, however, uncommon.

Causes

The brain has a greater requirement for oxygen and glucose fuel than any other part of the body. Oxygen and glucose are carried by the blood, and a continuous adequate supply of blood is essential for its continued function. Transient ischemic attacks occur when, for some reason, this supply is locally discontinued or is inadequate. The cause of this interruption to the supply is either a temporary blockage of an arterial branch by an abnormal particle of material being carried in the blood (an embolus), or an intermittent reduction in blood supply to part of the brain.

Emboli may be large enough to block off an arterial branch completely, and this will usually cause a TIA lasting for more than an hour. Commonly, emboli consist of a brief shower of cholesterol crystals or clumped blood platelets and these come from the linings of carotid or other arteries affected by atherosclerosis. The reason for intermittent reduction or stoppage of local blood supply in the absence of embolism is not well understood, but it occurs in vessels narrowed by atherosclerosis. Complete blockage of a substantial

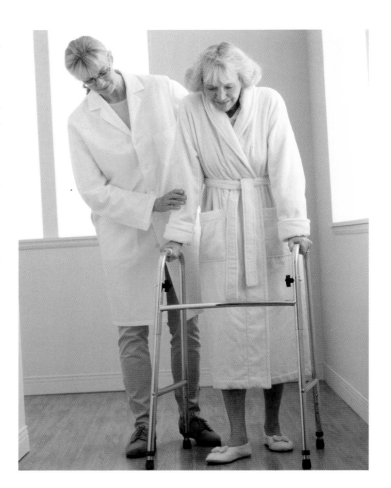

▲ *TIAs should be treated seriously, as they can lead to a stroke that may leave the patient with long-term disabilities.*

arterial branch by a blood clot that forms on a patch of atherosclerosis is called a cerebral thrombosis—the most common kind of stroke.

A TIA lasting for several hours suggests that an actual permanent blockage has occurred but that neighboring vessels have been able to open up sufficiently to maintain function. Even so, it is likely that some permanent damage to brain function has occurred. In some cases, repeated ischemic attacks of this kind lead to progressive loss of function. When this deterioration is rapid, the condition is known as stroke in evolution.

Treatment

The objective in treating any person who is having TIAs is to prevent stroke. A small daily dose of aspirin, which limits the aggregation of platelets and the formation of blood clots, can reduce the risk of stroke by about 13 percent. And the risk can be reduced further by adding a small dose of dipyramidol. Various other drugs have been shown to be similarly effective. Tissue plasminogen activator drugs, given early, can reverse the formation of blood clots. Blood pressure must be monitored and, if raised, controlled (see Blood Pressure).

Prevention is always better than treatment, and the best way of preventing TIAs and strokes is knowledge of the causes of atherosclerosis, and the avoidance of these causes by healthy living.

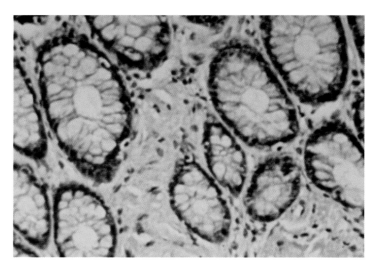

▲ *Cholesterol crystals in the blood can form an embolus that blocks off an artery, causing a transient ischemic attack.*

> *See also:* **Brain damage and disease; Stroke; Thrombosis**

Transplants

Questions and Answers

Can someone who has had a heart transplant be given another one if this fails or is rejected?

This has been attempted, but there are many problems involved. The rejection of a transplanted heart is often sudden and a further donor heart has to be available at very short notice, which is usually not the case. In addition, a second operation is much more difficult because there is always the problem that rejection can occur more quickly with the second operation. In the case of kidney replacements, however, repeated transplantation happens fairly often, since the patient can be maintained on a kidney machine until an organ becomes available.

My father, who is past retirement age, has bad heart trouble and his medication doesn't work well anymore. Would he be a candidate for a heart transplant?

Very few people are suitable for heart transplantation. The reason for this is that after a long period of heart disease, the lungs and other organs suffer damage; therefore, replacing the heart will not be enough to cure the problem. In general, heart transplants are performed on those whose heart failure is recent but so severe that it is clear that survival is not otherwise possible.

Is it possible to perform a brain transplant, and has it been tried?

To transplant the brain really means to perform a body transplant, since it is the brain that makes each of us an individual. This is not feasible now, nor is it likely to be, since all the nerves would stop functioning irreversibly once cut. The whole spinal cord would have to be transplanted as well, making this an inconceivable technical feat.

Not so long ago the idea of successfully transplanting an organ would have been considered pure science fiction. Today the number of people who have been given a new lease on life by a transplant is rapidly increasing.

The idea of replacing diseased parts of the body with spares is quite old, but it has become a reality only in the last few decades. There are considerable problems that must be overcome before transplants can be done, including locating suitable replacements and resolving important ethical questions that might arise. Despite this, the field of transplant surgery is expanding, since it offers the hope of treating illnesses that must otherwise be disabling or fatal.

Important and valuable work also takes place in the transplanting of other body tissues. Corneal grafting (see Cornea), and bone marrow transplants (see Marrow and Transplants) can be counted among some of the most successful procedures in this field of medicine.

In theory, any organ of the body except the brain can be transplanted in surgery, but a consistent level of success has been achieved only in operations involving the kidneys, heart, and liver. Transplantation of a lobe of a liver from a living donor can be successful and, recently, the injection of donated liver cells has been shown to be valuable in children with liver disease. Heart and lung transplantation has become fairly frequent; and much experimental work on the transplantation of other organs, and even hands, has been undertaken, with variable results.

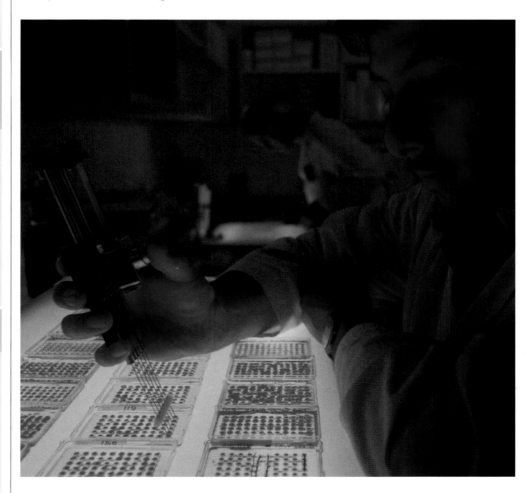

▲ *Before any transplant surgery can be performed, vital matching of both blood group and tissue type is carried out. Tissue types are found by testing white blood cells.*

Questions and Answers

Although heart transplants were considered experimental and very risky only two decades or so ago, 26,704 heart transplants have now been performed. Will they soon be considered a routine operation?

Transplants will certainly become more common as problems such as rejection and organ preservation for a pending transplantation are overcome. However, they may be just a stopgap in the history of spare part surgery, since it is likely that in the future synthetic organs will be designed. There would then be no problem of finding donors and the rejection that is inevitably associated with donor organs.

If I want to donate my body to medical research, can my relatives refuse to give their permission after my death?

No. If a person has expressed a positive wish to donate his or her organs in a will, by carrying a donor card, or by stating the intention in the presence of two witnesses during the last illness, then the relatives have no legal right to be consulted after the death. However, when death takes place in the hospital and the medical examiner wants to perform an autopsy, no part of the body can be removed without the medical examiner's permission.

I have heard that some people have had pancreas transplants to treat their diabetes. Is this true, and were the operations usually successful?

Pancreas transplants for diabetics have been mainly limited to patients who have kidney failure due to diabetes, because a person with a transplanted pancreas must remain on antirejection drugs indefinitely. If, however, this is required because the patient has to have a kidney transplant, the additional benefit of a fully functional pancreas and the cure of the diabetes can both be achieved at no extra disadvantage to the patient.

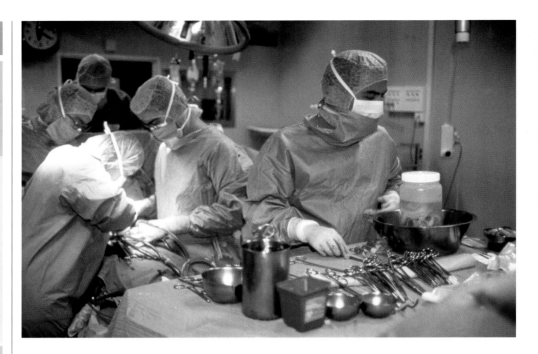

▲ *Surgeons perform a heart transplant on a patient. This type of surgery requires more than one surgeon; it is intricate and can take several hours to accomplish.*

Physical and ethical problems

Finding donor organs to transplant into patients who depend on them for continued life is one of the most difficult of the immediate problems that a surgeon has to face.

The organ should come from a person who was fit and preferably young at the time of his or her death. The tragedy of modern living is that the most likely way for this to occur is through a traffic accident.

Great care must be taken to ensure that the organs are removed only after death has occurred. At the same time, however, the organ to be used in a transplant will deteriorate quite quickly if it is no longer supplied with blood after death. Therefore it must be removed as soon as possible. It is this dilemma that has provoked most controversy in recent years because it was rapidly discovered that the exact point of death was more difficult to define than to recognize.

The solution to this problem centered on whether the brain was alive in the sense of being capable of recovering independent life support. After careful study of the survival of many victims of brain damage there have now emerged clear-cut ways in which doctors can determine the point at which brain death has occurred (see Brain).

Once brain death has been confirmed, the organ for transplant can be removed immediately after the respirator has been switched off. Although this can seem macabre, the reality is no more unpleasant than the death of a victim in other circumstances.

There is a crucial shortage of available organs, particularly where kidney transplants are concerned. This is because of the difficulty of coordinating the teams of surgeons doing the transplant, and the doctors caring for the trauma victim.

When an organ has been taken from a dead donor it must be preserved until it can be placed in the recipient. The organ must be placed on ice and special fluid pumped through its blood vessel system to keep the system open and free of blood clots. The technology required during this crucial period is being constantly updated and in the case of kidneys is quite advanced. The kidney is simply flushed through to remove the blood. It is then put into a polyethylene bag that is surrounded by ice. It can be kept in this state for up to 36 hours before being used.

Living donor transplants

Transplants from living donors are common in kidney transplantation, since a normal person can easily survive in good health with only one kidney. If a relative is prepared to give one of his or her kidneys, this is often the best match, since it lessens the risk of rejection. A close relative such as a brother, sister, or parent will share many genetic characteristics of the recipient; there is thus

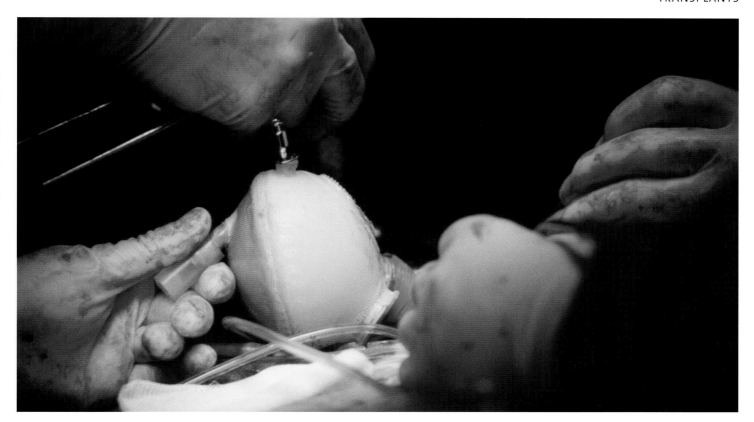

a chance that the recipient's immune system will not recognize the graft as foreign and reject it. The kidney for transplantation can be removed calmly without the urgency that is called for in a recently dead donor, allowing more time to plan the operation (see Donors).

Rejection of the transplant

Rejection is the main problem of transplant surgery, and directly or indirectly leads to most of the failures that occur. The body has a powerful defense system designed to repel the invasion of its domains by bacteria and viruses. The invaders are recognized because their chemicals are subtly different from those of our body. Unfortunately when a transplanted organ comes into contact with the body cells that act as soldiers in this defense force (see Immune System), the chemical makeup of the transplant is recognized as foreign and a reaction is mounted against it as though it were a host of bacteria (see Bacteria).

For this reason attempts are made before transplant surgery to match the type of tissue of the donor organ and the recipient. This is similar to blood grouping, since everyone has a tissue type as well as a blood group. Tissue types are discovered by testing the white blood cells; blood groups reflect the chemical makeup of the more numerous red blood cells (see Blood; Blood Groups).

Apart from trying to match the blood group and tissue type of the donor organ with that of the patient receiving it, there are various things that can be done to stop rejection. For example, it has been discovered that the more transfusions a patient has prior to surgery, the less likely he or she is to reject the transplant (see Blood Transfusion). This preventive effect occurs because the body's immune system is confronted many times with foreign tissues of donated blood. It seems to become more tolerant of other invasions and less likely to reject a transplanted organ. More deliberate

▲ *At the University of Utah in Salt Lake City, surgeons transplant an artificial heart into a calf.*

prevention takes the form of using powerful drugs to control the immune system so it cannot mount its attack on the new organ. This is a double-edged sword, since the body needs some immunity to fight against infecting bacteria, viruses, or fungi (see Infection and Infectious Diseases). The development of the drug cyclosporin was a major breakthrough. This drug selectively discourages rejection of tissue without unduly interfering with the other protective functions of the immune system.

Other complications

Apart from the complications caused by the drugs used in preventing rejection, other problems can arise. These include surgical problems that are related to the considerable task of sewing the organ in place. The blood vessels into the transplant must be carefully joined to prevent bleeding once the circulation is reestablished. Similarly, in the case of the kidney, the tubes carrying urine from the transplant must be delicately sewn into the recipient's bladder; and in a liver transplant, bile ducts must be implanted into the intestine.

The surgery

Usually, with the kidneys or the liver, the whole of the organ is transplanted into the patient's body, although segmental liver grafts can be performed from a live donor. The liver is placed similarly to its normal position, though the arteries used to supply it with blood are changed by grafting them to nearby intestinal arteries.

It is difficult to insert a new kidney in the position of the diseased one, which is usually left where it is. The new kidney is placed in the

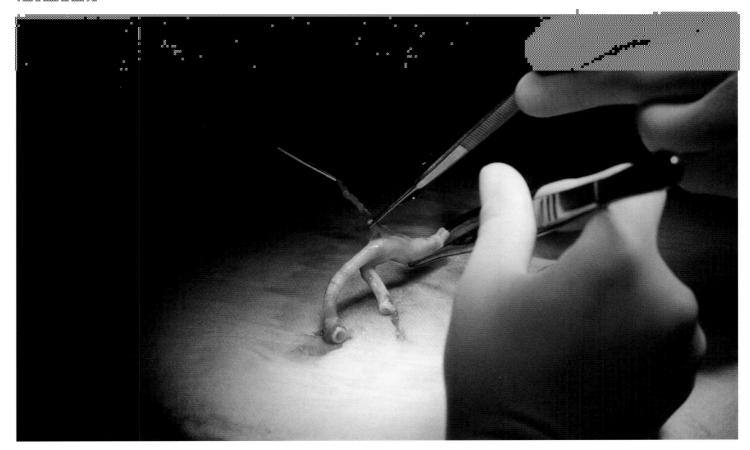

pelvis, which is conveniently spacious; this allows the new kidney's blood vessels to be joined to the large vessels to and from the legs. Another consideration is that in this position the joining of the ureter, the tube that carries urine to the bladder of the recipient, is made far easier (see Kidneys and Kidney Diseases; Kidney Transplants). When a heart is transplanted the whole of the diseased

▼ *Tissue expanders, traditionally used in plastic surgery, are to be used under the skin in pioneering transplant surgery.*

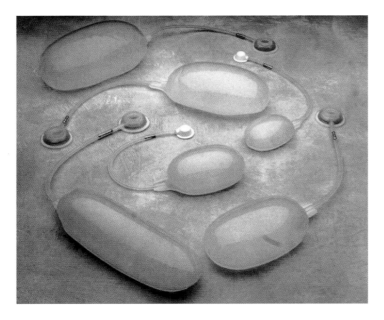

▲ *Surgeons prepare a section of artery for use in a liver transplant operation. The artery being used comes from the dead victim of an automobile accident.*

heart is not removed. This is both unnecessary and unnecessarily complicating. Two large veins enter the right upper chamber and four large veins enter the left upper chamber of the heart. Because of this, the greater part of the two upper chambers of the patient's own heart is commonly left in place so that six fewer major blood vessels have to be connected. It is usually the lower chambers, the ventricles, that are severely diseased and it these that are replaced by the donor heart, leaving only two large arteries to be reconnected (see Heart Transplants).

Postoperative care

After any surgery there is a risk of infection, but the recipient of a transplant is at particular risk. Measures are taken to protect the patients from germs, by isolating them in a special room, or people attending them and visiting them wear special clothing and masks—or both measures may be taken. Acute rejection is a risk a few days after the operation, and even after this there may be a risk of chronic rejection, which is slower in causing the loss of the organ but equally dangerous. Once the drugs suppressing the rejection process start to work, the person may gradually return to a fairly normal life. In the case of many kidney transplants, the recipients can return to work, and many women who have had a kidney transplant have given birth to healthy children.

See also: Stroke; Surgery

Trauma center

Patients suffering from severe and possibly life-threatening injuries will be admitted to a trauma center. Such centers have a specialized team of surgeons and medical practitioners who have access to surgical and life-support equipment for 24 hours a day, seven days a week.

Trauma centers are specialized hospital facilities that diagnose and treat patients with severe injuries. The aim of these centers is to quickly respond and treat traumatic injury through a multidisciplinary team of health professionals. Close coordination with the emergency medical services (EMS) is also important. Trauma injuries are the most common cause of death in children and young adults in the United States, with over 100,000 fatalities a year. Although millions of Americans survive their injuries, many are left with long-term disabilities. Motor vehicle collisions, falls, gun wounds, knife wounds, and farm accidents are all common causes of serious injury.

History

An organized system to treat severely injured patients was first developed by the American military when treating soldiers wounded in World War II. These systems were refined in the Korean and Vietnam wars, with developments that included specialized field hospitals for traumatic injuries. Because of the success of these military hospitals, the civilian population in the United States wanted similar facilities in public hospitals. The first of these trauma centers were created in urban municipal hospitals that gave emergency services to people without health insurance.

A number of reports and government acts followed to shape the current U.S. trauma care system. In particular, an influential document by the National Academy of Sciences (NAS), "Accidental Death and Disability: The Neglected Disease of Modern Society" (1966) gave further motivation for a widespread trauma and emergency medical service. Through the 1970s a large amount of government funds helped form an infrastructure of around 300 emergency medical service and trauma centers nationwide. This funding declined in the 1980s and 1990s, with a

How many trauma centers does the United States have?

A recent survey by Bishops and Associates, a leading organization in trauma center development, listed 747 trauma centers in the United States. These centers are divided into levels that describe how advanced they are. There are 214 of the most sophisticated centers having level I facilities such as research and teaching; 406 level II centers that give full round-the-clock trauma care; 97 less advanced level III facilities, usually consisting of the emergency medical services and a team of surgeons; and 30 others that are not graded.

What are the most common injuries treated by a trauma center?

The National Trauma Data Bank states that the most common causes of severe injury are motor vehicle collisions (about 40 percent of cases), followed by falls (28 percent), then gunshot wounds (8 percent). Of these, the number of fatalities were about 4 percent of cases for motor vehicle collisions, about 3 percent of falls, and almost 9 percent of gunshot wounds. About another 10 percent of injuries were also vehicle-related, involving motorcycles, bicycles, and injuries to pedestrians.

How are trauma centers funded?

The large costs of funding a trauma center usually fall on the hospital. This can discourage hospitals from developing trauma center facilities. A few state initiatives help pay for some trauma costs. Certain states, such as Illinois and Washington, use revenues from traffic fines. They say this is because motor vehicles are the largest cause of injury. Other states use a portion of their tobacco settlement funds. Some states are seeking to tax firearms or use fines from illegal use of guns.

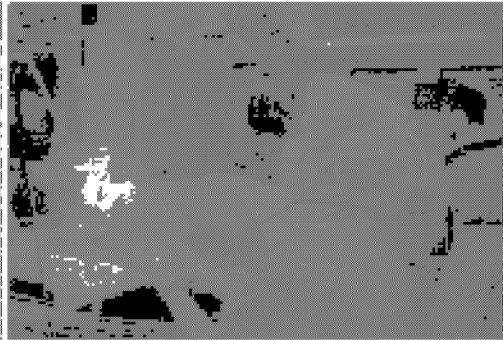

▲ *A trauma patient who was a victim of a violent crime is receiving medical treatment in the emergency department of a hospital in Washington, D.C.*

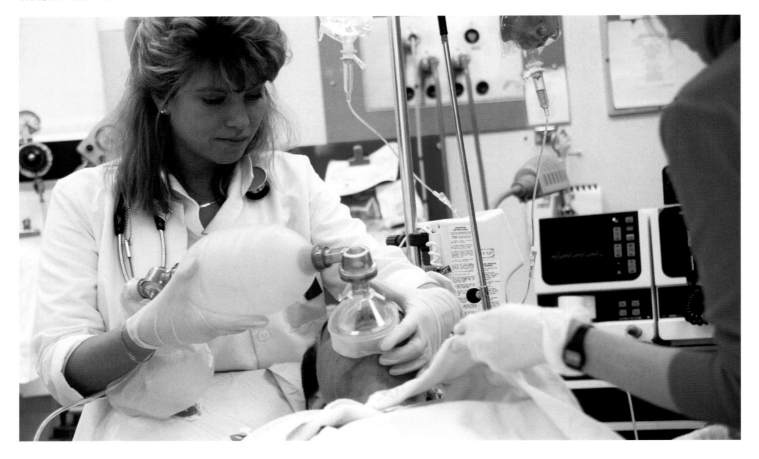

▲ *A nurse fits a respiration bag on a trauma patient to help him breathe while his body copes with the loss of blood.*

corresponding fall in patient care. In 1999 a report from the Institute of Medicine (IOM) said that while there had been significant advances in trauma care, too little funding was being invested in tackling the problems of treating injuries (see Health Care System).

Trauma care systems

A trauma care system is an organized set of facilities to make sure that severely injured patients receive the best and most efficient medical care. It encompasses the emergency medical services, the trauma center, and a rehabilitation process to improve the patient's recovery after the injury. Injury prevention schemes such as safety legislation regarding seat belts and public education about smoke detectors are also an important part of a good trauma care system.

The first stage of a full trauma care system is to make sure an injured person is quickly reached by the emergency medical services. The patient should have the necessary treatment at the scene, and then be rapidly taken to the closest and most appropriate trauma center to receive surgical and medical care. For victims of severe injuries, the time taken to reach a trauma center will often determine whether they live or die, with the first hour—the so-called "golden hour"—being the most crucial period.

Before treatment can begin the patient must undergo triage, which is the method of sorting injured patients by the urgency of their need for treatment. Part of this process is carried out by the emergency medical services, which assess the injury and decide on the most appropriate trauma center. At the center, patients are then allocated the relevant medical resources for their condition—for example, they might need to be placed in a burns unit or see a specialist in spinal injury (see Burn Center).

The trauma center is staffed by a multidisciplinary trauma team, which consists of a group of health professionals who together treat and manage the injured patients. This team includes trauma surgeons, emergency medicine physicians, anesthesiologists, radiologists, and specialized nurses. These professionals have access to a specially designed range of equipment and facilities, including an inpatient trauma care unit, surgery suites, and possibly a burn center. In addition, there may be other specialized units and teams, such as a pediatric intensive care unit for severely injured children, or specialized surgeons for treating brain or spinal injuries.

Many trauma centers also have a rehabilitation team to help patients come to terms with and manage their injuries. Rehabilitation is the process by which physical, sensory, and mental capabilities are restored or redeveloped after damage. Appropriate rehabilitation reduces the time spent in a hospital and improves a patient's chances of a successful recovery (see Rehabilitation).

Costs

In 1995, for example, the medical cost of injury in the United States was about $260 billion, which constituted about 12 percent of all health spending. Further, this amount did not include the economic costs, such as lost working hours, or quality-of-life factors. The emotional and financial impact on victims of severe trauma can be terrible, both to themselves and their family and friends. For example, many trauma victims can be disabled by their injuries for the rest of their lives (see Handicaps).

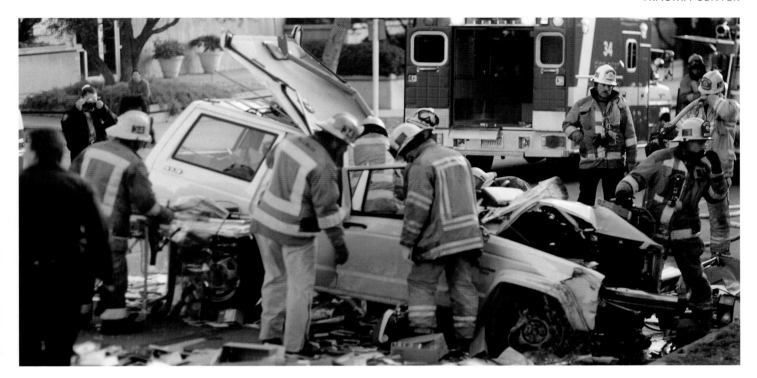

Problems

Although there is much evidence to show that trauma care saves lives, for most people their treatment will be either disorganized or unavailable. This poor treatment results in unnecessary death and disability for thousands every year. Some reports estimate that almost 35 percent of all trauma deaths occur from a lack of appropriate care. Because these deficiencies depend on where a patient lives they can affect anyone, rich or poor, irrespective of his or her health insurance.

There is a broad agreement in the trauma care community that the government needs to take action to reduce death and disability from serious injury. These trauma experts say the first step should be to create a national body to implement the legislation and funding of an

▲ *Victims of car accidents account for about 40 percent of the trauma cases in U.S. hospitals.*

important government trauma act dating from 1990. Spending on this act was blocked by Congress in 1995 and since then has received only sporadic funding. Completing this act should aid the millions of Americans injured every year, and also help hospitals to be better prepared for mass casualty situations such as acts of terrorism.

The future

Experts suggest several ways of improving the current system of trauma care. The causes and treatment of traumatic injury are well known, as with other ailments such as cancer and heart disease. Therefore, trauma should be preventable in many cases, and there are also many suggestions for improving existing treatments.

A main focus of trauma care in the future will be to make greater use of injury prevention schemes to stop potential trauma before it happens. At present, injury prevention initiatives vary widely from state to state. In the future, experts imagine each state as having a core injury prevention program. Further, data from a central trauma registry will help identify particular causes of injury to act or legislate against.

Another aspect of trauma care that could be improved in the future is the distribution of trauma centers across the country. For example, hospitals might use innovative methods such as mobile trauma units in rural areas. Furthermore, linking trauma systems through computer networks would make treatments more efficient and effective. The creation of a national trauma database would allow trauma care to be directed at the areas in most need, while giving researchers valuable data for improving existing trauma systems (see Medical Information Highway).

Types of trauma centers
There are several levels of trauma center, with level I being the most advanced and level V the most basic. The following categories are defined by the American College of Surgeons.
Level I: Full range of services with research and teaching.
Level II: Full range of services.
Level III: Availability of a general surgeon and orthopedic, neurosurgical (for brain injuries), and emergency services for 24 hours a day.
Level IV: Emergency services and an available surgeon.
Level V: A non-physician-staffed clinic, for example an emergency care facility with an advanced nurse practitioner. These are found only in Washington state.

See also: Critical care unit; Emergency department; Hospitals; Intensive care unit;

Travel and health

Questions and Answers

I am going on vacation to Europe. Is it possible I could catch rabies?

Although rare, rabies still exists in eastern Europe, especially in the Baltic countries and Turkey, so keep away from strays and wild animals. Rabies can be transmitted by a lick, bite, or scratch from an infected animal. If you are scratched or bitten, wash the wound promptly with soap and clean water and, if you can, apply alcohol. Then go to the nearest hospital or doctor as quickly as possible so that you can be given a rabies vaccination if it is considered necessary.

When I go on vacation I often suffer from heat exhaustion. What causes this, and how can I avoid it?

This is caused by excessive loss of fluid and salt from the circulation by sweating. Keep out of the midday sun, drink plenty of water, and take salt tablets to replace the salt you lose when you sweat. Excessive unprotected exposure to high temperatures may lead to heatstroke, which is a serious and potentially fatal condition.

I have an allergy to a particular antibiotic. How can I make sure I am not given this if I am taken seriously ill while on vacation?

If you have an allergy or a reaction to a certain medicine you should wear a medical alert bracelet. In the event of illness or an accident in which you become unconscious, this will warn anyone treating you.

If I need an injection while I am abroad, how will I know whether the needle is sterile?

In some poorer countries sterile needles are a rarity, so you should take an emergency pack with you that contains sterilized syringes, needles, drip needles, dressings, swabs, and suture materials.

Traveling at home or abroad presents all kinds of health risks, from motion sickness to malaria. There are a number of simple measures people can take to ensure that their trips are not ruined by an avoidable health problem.

Travel can all too often be ruined because people fail to take the necessary health precautions before and during the trip. For traveling at home or abroad, there are some basic guidelines to follow that will reduce the risk of illness and lessen the strain of long journeys.

It is a good idea for people to find out as much as possible about the country or place they are visiting before they go. The best sources of information are the Internet, travel agents, the embassy or tourist office, or the airline if people are traveling by air. The Department of State publishes useful "Background Notes" on about 170 countries worldwide. These are brief factual pamphlets giving information on each country.

Packing for comfort

Once the destination has been decided upon, the weather conditions that are likely to be experienced during the visit need to be investigated so that the appropriate clothing can be brought. For example, if the weather is likely to be hot, then it is sensible to avoid wearing clothes that are made of nonabsorbent materials, such as nylon or polyester, next to the skin.

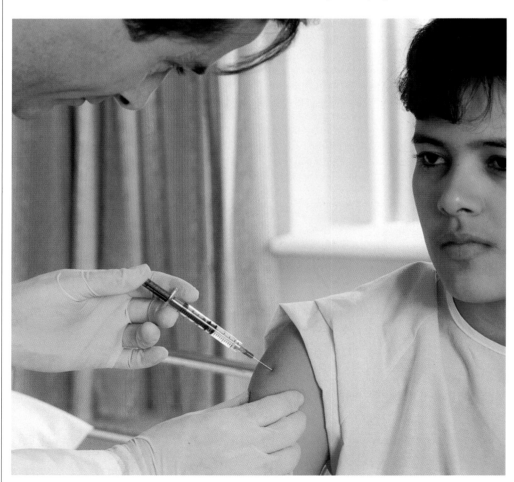

▲ *If a person is traveling overseas and needs to have a course of vaccinations, these should be arranged with a doctor or hospital clinic well in advance.*

These synthetic materials do not soak up perspiration and will leave the skin feeling cold and clammy; prickly heat and, in the case of footwear, athlete's foot may then result. Natural fibers (such as cotton) are absorbent and therefore more comfortable and less likely to cause skin problems (see Athlete's Foot; Prickly Heat). For travel overseas to a hot climate, lightweight clothes in light colors that will reflect the heat are best, rather than clothing in dark colors that will absorb it and retain the heat.

If a person is going to a very cold climate he or she will need to wear clothes that will prevent frostbite. These should include warm outdoor clothes, gloves, thick socks, and a hat that covers both the head and the ears (see Frostbite).

Wherever a traveler is going, it is important to wear loose, comfortable clothes for the journey so that there is nothing to impede the blood flow or the circulation of air around the body. Your feet may swell if you have to sit for a long period in an airplane, bus, automobile, or train, so it is best to travel in comfortable shoes.

Although most forms of transport are air-conditioned and comfortable, there may be a risk of dehydration, especially on long flights, so avoid consuming alcohol, and drink plenty of mineral water or soft drinks while traveling.

Motion sickness

Most people are unlikely to be airsick, unless there is a great deal of turbulence, but for some people long automobile, bus, or train journeys can lead to motion sickness. People who suffer from motion sickness should try sitting in the front of the vehicle and keep their eyes on the route ahead. They should also avoid eating fatty foods or having a large meal before traveling, since these sit heavily in the stomach. Eating crystallized ginger or taking ginger capsules before setting off, and sucking candy or cough drops during the journey, can help. Acupressure on the forearm, two thumb-widths above the center of the wrist, can also help reduce symptoms.

If traveling by ship, the traveler should stay on deck, especially if the sea is rough. It will help to keep the eyes on the horizon. A doctor will be able to recommend seasickness drugs, but these often cause drowsiness, so they should be avoided if a traveler is planning to drive once he or she disembarks. To be effective, motion sickness medication such as promethazine should be taken about an hour before the journey begins, then every 12 hours as required. Acupressure may help to relieve nausea (see Acupressure).

Vaccinations

Vaccinations need to be considered well in advance of any overseas travel because some involve a course of treatment that has to be given at monthly intervals. Vaccinations for international travel can be grouped into three basic categories: those necessary for entry; those that all travelers have as a matter of course; and those for protection against specific diseases associated with the area the traveler intends to visit. Under the International Health Regulations, cholera and yellow fever are the only two vaccinations that may be required on entry.

▼ *Most people take out insurance to cover the theft of personal possessions while overseas, but you should also remember to take out good medical insurance.*

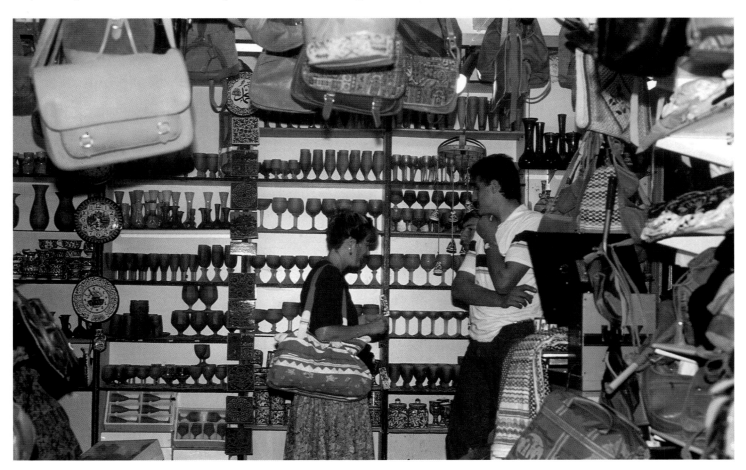

Since the current cholera vaccine is only about 50 percent effective, the World Health Organization (WHO) discourages countries from upholding policies that require cholera vaccination for entry. However, in some developing countries, especially in Africa, proof of cholera vaccination may still need to be shown. This consists of a signed and validated International Certificate of Vaccination that is dated not less than six days, or more than six months, prior to the visitor's arrival in the country. This is because the vaccine's protection lasts only six months. It is sensible for a traveler to have the vaccination if he or she is planning to make an extended visit to a high-risk area where medical help may not be on hand, or if a doctor advises it for medical reasons.

Some countries will refuse visitors entry without an International Certificate of Vaccination for yellow fever. This is especially important if a visitor is returning from a country that is currently infected (see Infection and Infectious Diseases), even if he or she has not been to the actual area within the country that is affected. Visitors may also be asked for proof of vaccination if they have visited any countries where yellow fever is known to be a problem. The vaccine needs to be given at least ten days, but not more than ten years, before traveling.

Depending on the destination and the nature and duration of the stay, the traveler's doctor may suggest other vaccinations for diseases such as Japanese encephalitis, meningococcal meningitis, hepatitis A, typhoid, and rabies (see Encephalitis; Meningitis; Rabies).

Malaria

In many parts of Africa, Asia, and Central and South America, people can get malaria if they are bitten by an infected mosquito. Travelers need to find out whether malaria is prevalent where they are going, and if it is, they should arrange for a course of antimalarial pills.

There are different pills for different areas and to combat the many different strains of malaria. The pills need to be taken before the traveler sets off, while he or she is away, and for at least one month after the return. If the person feels ill or just generally poorly during the immediate weeks after returning home, it is advisable to go to a doctor and have a medical checkup.

Sun sense

Although the temptation to lie in the sun may be strong, it must be remembered that ultraviolet (UV) exposure causes aging and wrinkles, and there is a possibility that overexposure can lead to skin cancer (see Skin and Skin Diseases). Travelers should try to avoid being out in the

First-aid checklist

The following items cover basic first-aid requirements if you are traveling abroad. You also need to include any regular medication you are taking.

Motion sickness remedy
Antidiarrhea pills
Antiseptic cream
Salt pills
Calamine lotion
Insect repellent
Antimalarial pills
Sting relief or hydrocortisone preparation
Indigestion pills
Acetaminophen
Water purifying tablets
Scissors
Band-Aids
Cotton pads
Bandages
Contraceptives (if necessary)

middle of the day when the sun's rays are at their strongest, limit the time they spend in the sun, and be especially careful at the start of the stay.

Protection from the sun's rays can be achieved by covering up and using a high-factor sunscreen on any exposed skin; this screen is reapplied frequently, especially after swimming. The head should be covered with a sun hat, and sunglasses should be worn to protect the eyes. Some drugs, including tetracyclines and tranquilizers, actually increase the skin's sensitivity to the sun, so travelers should check with their doctors if they are taking these (see Tetracyclines; Tranquilizers). If a traveler does get sunburn, the skin should be soothed with calamine or aloe vera lotion, or calendula ointment, and he or she should stay out of the sun until the skin is fully back to normal (see Sunburn).

Bites

Bites from insects, such as mosquitoes, can lead to severe itching, and because antimalarial pills are not 100 percent effective, in some countries there may also be a risk of catching malaria. Travelers should sleep under a mosquito net if possible, or protect themselves by using an insect repellent spray. Slow-burning antimosquito coils can be used at night. If a traveler does get bitten, he or she should try not to scratch. Instead the bite should be treated with an antihistamine spray or cream, or soothed with calamine lotion.

In case of contact with a sea urchin or jellyfish, ammonia (sold in stick form) should be applied to relieve the sting.

Diarrhea and dysentery

One of the most common illnesses experienced by travelers is diarrhea, with attacks lasting from one to three days (see Diarrhea). Dysentery, a cause of serious diarrhea, is often accompanied by vomiting, fever, and abdominal pain, which may lead to serious dehydration.

Diarrhea is usually caused by bacteria present in contaminated water, milk, or food, although the change of environment, the climate, too much alcohol, and even dehydration can also cause it.

To avoid diarrhea, travelers should drink only bottled water or sterilize all drinking water, either by boiling it or with sterilizing tablets. They should not have ice in drinks and should always use sterilized water for brushing the teeth and washing any fruit or salads. Milk should be boiled unless it has been pasteurized, and high-risk foods, such as shellfish, raw or undercooked meat, egg products, and unwashed fruits and vegetables, should be avoided. As well as these basic precautions daily prophylactic pills that guard against stomach upsets should be taken.

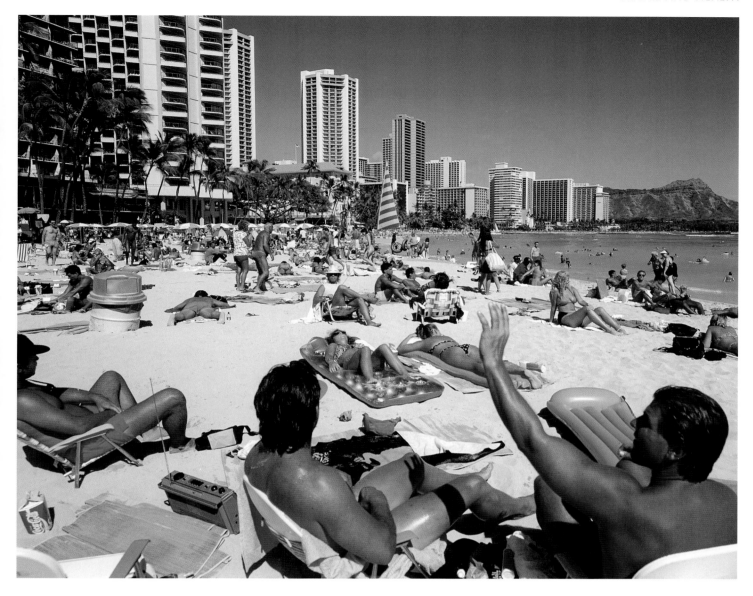

Safe sex

The only way to have safe sex, especially if it is casual sex, is by using a condom. Travelers should be able to buy condoms at their destination, but if they think they may be likely to need some, they should buy them before they set off. They should also not let the sun and alcohol go to their heads so that they forget this precaution against pregnancy and sexually transmitted diseases, including AIDS (see AIDS; Sexually Transmitted Diseases). Travelers should use a condom even if they or their new partners are taking the Pill.

Travelers should also remember that a prolonged bout of diarrhea or vomiting can reduce the effectiveness of the contraceptive pill (see Oral Contraceptives).

Medical insurance

The Social Security Medicare Program does not cover hospital or medical services outside the United States, so travelers will need to take out separate medical insurance against sickness and accident if they are traveling overseas. They should always check what the coverage includes, especially for sporting activities, and read any small print before traveling.

▲ *People who spend their vacations lying on the beach should wear plenty of sunscreen and limit their sun exposure time.*

There are a number of emergency medical assistance companies operating internationally that offer urgent medical treatment for their member travelers. A travel agent will be able to supply the necessary information about these companies.

On return

Sometimes illnesses can take a few weeks to develop, so a traveler may not actually become sick until after his or her return. If a traveler does become sick in the first few weeks after returning from an overseas trip, he or she should tell the doctor which countries were visited and what vaccinations or medications were taken before the visits or while he or she was away.

See also: **Bites and stings; Cholera; Dysentery; Hepatitis; Malaria; Motion sickness; Sunstroke; Tropical diseases; Typhoid and paratyphoid; Vaccinations; Yellow fever**

Tremor

I play the violin in the local orchestra and have been troubled by a tremor when performing in concerts. Can anything be done about this?

This is a common problem among musicians and other people who have to perform in public. Beta-blocking drugs that inhibit the effects of epinephrine can be used just before the performance. Consult your doctor because he or she will be able to advise you about this form of treatment.

Both my father and I have a marked shaking of the hands most of the time. Does it run in families? For example, will my son be similarly affected?

There is a tendency for tremor of this type to run in families and your son may be affected. It is called benign essential tremor and does not imply a serious neurological disorder.

I get very nervous in strange surroundings and can shake so badly that drinking is a problem. Is this abnormal?

No. It is normal to tremble when nervous, but your degree of nervousness may be excessive. Your doctor may feel that treatment would be useful.

My father has Parkinson's disease, and a tremor of the fingers worsens when he is anxious. Is it due to anxiety or the disease?

It depends on what the tremor looks like. The familiar rolling of the thumb and fingers that occurs in Parkinson's disease is easy to distinguish from the tremble of pure nervousness. However, even if your father's shake is due to his disease it will become much worse when he is nervous or attention is drawn to it.

Most people know what it feels like to tremble with fear or to be a bit unsteady after overindulgence and lack of sleep. However, sometimes a tremor can be an indication of a serious disorder of the nervous system.

Many people are familiar with the involuntary shaking in the hands that they experience when they are nervous or have had a bad shock. This is the most common type of tremor, and is experienced most commonly in the hands, feet, jaw, tongue, and head. In fact, everyone has a very slight tremor, even when relaxed or asleep, and this can be measured by sensitive instruments. It is called physiological tremor, and the noticeable shake that occurs under stress is simply an exaggeration of this.

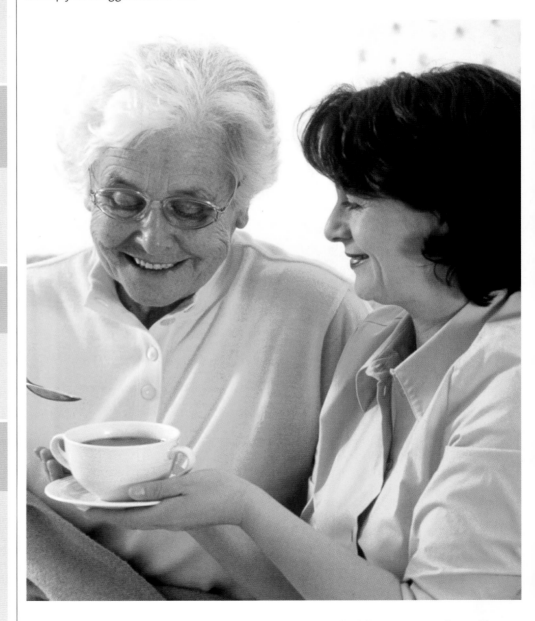

▲ *The simple act of taking a drink can turn into an ordeal for someone who suffers from a tremor. Asking for assistance can help a sufferer neatly overcome this problem.*

The body's natural physiological tremor is also exaggerated in certain diseases. The only difference is that it is present without any obvious anxiety. Other forms of shaking of the limbs, when a person is either at rest or in action, may look different. It is often possible to pinpoint from the characteristics of the tremor which area of the nervous system is damaged (see Nervous System).

What is tremor?

For any action to be smooth and unfaltering, or even for a hand or foot to be kept gently at rest, the muscles that move it must be balanced, each one contracting by just the right amount (see Muscles). Synchronization of different groups of muscles is coordinated at many different levels in the nervous system, particularly in the basal ganglia deep in the cerebral hemispheres, and in the cerebellum that bulges at the back of the brain stem. Even holding the hands still against the force of gravity is an active process, with messages being matched in the lifting and dropping groups of muscles.

Physiological tremor represents the minute oscillations in the different groups of muscles as they try to maintain this balance. If

▼ *The morning shakes after a night of heavy drinking can indicate alcohol dependence, and should make a drinker seriously consider regulating his or her alcohol intake.*

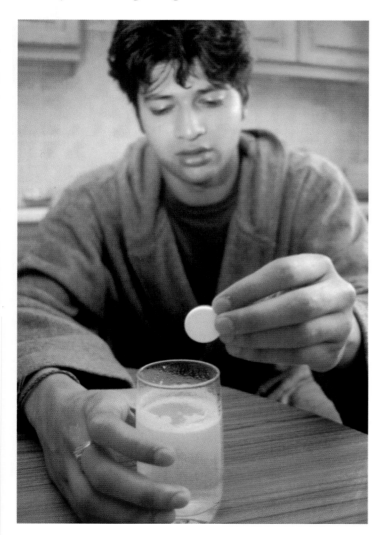

the functioning of the basal ganglia or cerebellum is disturbed, these main controllers of movement can no longer contribute fully to the delicate balancing act, and more pronounced movement swings occur (see Brain).

Common types of tremor

The most common tremors are those that are an exaggeration of normal physiological tremor. The most common cause is anxiety or nervousness; in this case the tremor is caused mainly by an excess of the chemical epinephrine that courses through the blood during anxiety states. The extra chemical has the effect of increasing the swings of movement in the muscles, making them easily visible.

Other causes of this type of tremor are an overactive thyroid gland (see Thyroid) and alcohol addiction (see Alcoholism). In some families there is a tendency to an exaggeration of the normal physiological tremor. This is called benign essential tremor, and is not an indication of any disease. Similarly, the slight persistent tremor that is commonly experienced by older people does not indicate any disease.

Other types of tremor

A more disabling form of tremor happens in people who have damage to the cerebellum or its major connections in the brain stem. This condition is called intention tremor, since it appears only when an intentional movement is made. The movement is broken up by increasingly wild oscillations, and is a disabling characteristic of advanced multiple sclerosis (see Multiple Sclerosis).

A typical shaking of the fingers when a person is at rest occurs commonly in Parkinson's disease. This used to be called pill-rolling tremor, since the affected person seems to be always rolling a ball between the thumb and first two fingers (see Parkinson's Disease). The shaking disappears when a voluntary action is made, and the main disability it causes is embarrassment. This type of shaking, as with the intention tremor, is made far worse by anxiety (see Anxiety).

A mixture of intention tremor and pill-rolling tremor occurs with damage to a particular collection (nucleus) of brain cells, and is known as red nucleus tremor. The most common cause of this type of tremor is multiple sclerosis.

A different type of shaking is seen when there is failure of the kidneys or liver, with a consequent derangement of the body's metabolism. For a split second, all muscle activity ceases and then returns just as quickly. Thus an outstretched hand may appear to flap if a person tries to keep it outstretched (see Kidneys and Kidney Diseases; Liver and Liver Diseases).

Tremor can also be provoked by such drugs as antidepressant and antipsychotic drugs and caffeine.

Can tremor be treated?

Depending on the type of tremor, there is often a good chance of treatment. Exaggerated physiological tremor can be improved by drugs that suppress the nervous system. Drugs to combat Parkinson's disease can improve a tremor, but often have more effect on the other aspects of this disorder. Intention tremor, as seen in multiple sclerosis, is very difficult to treat, but because of the natural waxing and waning of the disease, this problem may not persist.

See also: **Epilepsy; Side effects; Withdrawal symptoms**

2275

Trichinosis

Questions and Answers

Could I catch trichinosis in this country or only in the tropics?

You certainly could get it in this country. In fact, it is rare in the tropics but common in America and Europe. Infection occurs through eating pork that is infected, so it is most common in those countries where a lot of pork is eaten.

There was evidence of trichinosis on my chest X ray, but I haven't been sick. Could I have had the disease without knowing it?

Yes. It is common to have the disease without being aware of it. The reason why abnormalities are seen on X rays is that the larvae form cysts in the muscles that protect them for up to two years; eventually, however, the cysts become calcified (impregnated with chalk), and this calcification shows up on an X ray. Studies done in the United States on muscle samples taken at autopsy have shown some evidence of infection in 20 percent of cases. The figure for the UK is nearer to 1 percent.

Can trichinosis be prevented?

Yes. One of the most effective ways of preventing it is not to eat pork. This has been practiced for centuries according to religious custom by Jews, Muslims, and Hindus. In societies where pork is eaten, preventive measures are to freeze meat before cooking, or to cook it thoroughly. Irradiation of pork using radioactive cobalt or cesium has also been used. Another preventive measure is to take proper care when raising hogs. Uncooked hog swill may contain infected raw scraps or even feces from an infected animal; this leads to the spread of infection. The disease is fairly widespread among animals like rats, and this is a source of infection, since hogs sometimes kill rats.

Trichinosis, one of the most common worm infections in human beings, can be a serious illness. Prevention is simple, however, and consists mainly in ensuring that pork, which contains the parasite, is always properly cooked.

Trichinosis is most common in Europe and in North America and is fairly uncommon in the tropics. It does not occur in Australia or in the islands of the Pacific.

Cause

The illness is caused by a small worm, called *Trichinella spiralis*, which may infest all meat-eating creatures. It lives in the intestine in its adult form, and male and female worms mate to produce huge numbers of larvae. These then spread through the bloodstream to the muscles, where they form protective cysts in which they can survive for a long period. In the meantime, the adult

HOW TRICHINOSIS OCCURS

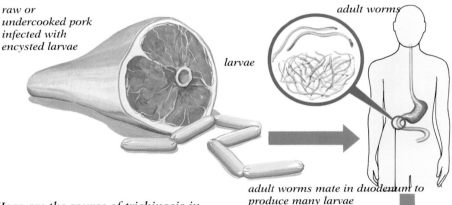

raw or undercooked pork infected with encysted larvae

larvae

adult worms

adult worms mate in duodenum to produce many larvae

larvae enter bloodstream, usually via the hepatic portal vein, and commonly settle in the heart, brain, and eyes

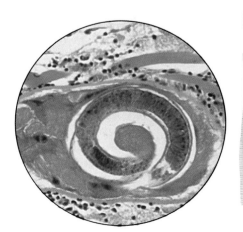

Hogs are the source of trichinosis in man. The larvae of the worm Trichinella spiralis *form protective cysts in the muscles of the hog, and if infected pork is eaten, the larvae are released, mature, and breed. The new larvae circulate around the body until they reach muscles in which to lodge. Infected hog swill (feed) perpetuates the cycle.*

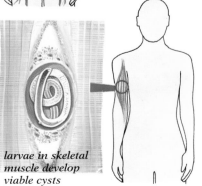

larvae in skeletal muscle develop viable cysts

worms in the intestines die. Each female probably lives about four to eight weeks, and during this time will produce about 1,500 larvae. The infection of the next host will occur if the original animal is caught and eaten by a predator. The muscles are eaten, cysts around the larvae dissolve, and new adults develop in the next host.

When the infecting larvae enter the duodenum of the new host, they work their way through the wall of the intestine and pass through four developmental stages before becoming adult males or females. The mature worms then return to the lumen (central space) of the intestine. As adult worms they are just visible. The male is 0.06 inch (1.6 mm) long and the female is 0.16 inch (4 mm) long. The male has a testis and the female has an ovary and a coiled tubular womb. Mating takes place as soon as two adult worms are present in the lumen of the intestine, and the female then starts to produce larvae. Once a larva is produced, it passes into the bloodstream and can come to rest in the muscles or any other part of the body. The most common sites include the heart, brain, and eye, as well as the ordinary muscles that the parasite is seeking. It is only the larvae that find muscle and form a protective cyst; the larvae that infest other organs soon disintegrate.

The main strain of the parasite is found in humans and in hogs, dogs, rats, and cats. The main source of infection is therefore pork, as far as human beings are concerned. The habit of eating uncooked pork sausages is particularly dangerous and infection runs very high in Germany and in countries, such as the United States, which have a strong German influence.

A second important biological strain is found in Arctic regions, and here the typical hosts are whales, walruses, seals, squirrels, foxes, and dogs. Bears, particularly polar bears, are very likely to become infected, being the most powerful predators in the Arctic.

Symptoms

Most cases of trichinosis occur without any visible external signs of infection, and they are discovered only by examining autopsy muscle samples under a microscope. There is evidence to suggest that up to 20 percent of the people in the United States, and 1 percent of people

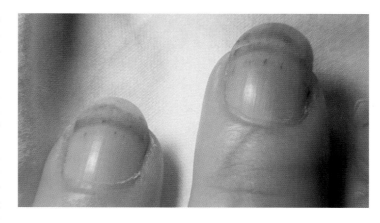

▲ *Splinter hemorrhages under the fingernails are indicative of the parasitic disease trichinosis.*

in the UK, have some degree of infection. Cysts in the muscles can also be seen on X-ray film as a result of calcification after about two years (see Muscles; X Rays).

Symptoms that occur indicate a very heavy infection. Diarrhea and vomiting may result when larvae invade the walls of the intestine, and this invasion may also provoke an allergic rash on the trunk and extremities. The major symptoms, of which there are four, appear when the larvae leave the intestine and start to circulate around the body. There will be fever; swelling of the eyelids and of the tissue around the eyes; pain in the muscles, which can be very severe; and a high level of eosinophils (a type of white blood cell) in the blood. Heart failure may develop if many larvae invade the heart.

By the third stage of the disease, when the larvae are forming cysts in the muscles, the patient may become very weak, and death may occur simply through exhaustion and poor nutrition. The brain can also become severely affected and various neurological complications may also manifest themselves. In serious infections, the fever will recede first, with the muscular pains persisting for some time. However, there is always the possibility of a secondary problem that will prove fatal.

Treatment and prevention

If the full-blown disease develops, steroid drugs are given to control the effects of the inflammation caused by the larvae (see Inflammation; Steroids). A drug called thiabendazole will kill the adult worms and is given to prevent the production of new larvae, although the larvae themselves cannot be killed.

Prevention consists in the proper preparation of pork, particularly with adequate cooking, and in reducing the risks of hogs' becoming infected.

See also: Fevers; Hookworms; Hygiene; Infection and infectious diseases; Parasites; Rashes; Symptoms; Worms

▼ *Trichinosis can be prevented by the proper care of hogs, particularly by ensuring that their food is free from contamination.*

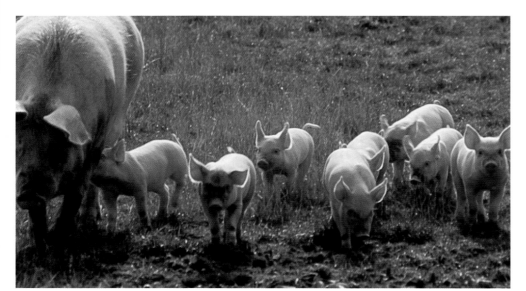

Trichomoniasis

Trichomoniasis is a common and highly infectious genital tract condition. The symptoms are both irritating and unpleasant, but fortunately this condition responds well to treatment.

Trichomoniasis is a common condition, with at least one in five women likely to have it at some time during life. It can affect men, being responsible for about 4 percent of cases of nonspecific urethritis, but more usually gives rise to disease in women, for whom it is among the most common causes of vaginal discharge (see Vagina; Vaginal Discharge).

Causes

The trichomonas organism, *Trichomonas vaginalis*, responsible for the infection is rather unusual. It is neither a bacterium nor a virus, but a single-cell, pear-shaped protozoan or parasite. Its five whiplike tentacles enable it both to swim about in the vaginal secretion and to attract particles of material on which it lives (see Protozoal Infections).

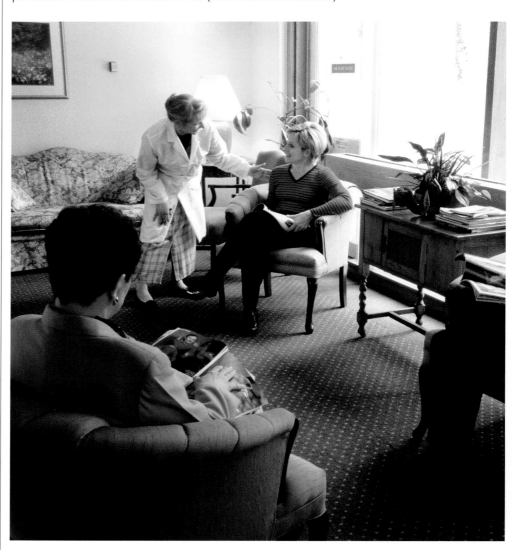

▲ *Trichomoniasis can be fully investigated at a special treatment center, which provides expert but informal medical care.*

Questions and Answers

I have an unpleasant vaginal discharge that seems like a trichomonas infection. Can I get rid of it myself by douching?

No; you should only take the drug required for the specific germ causing your vaginitis. This depends on identification of the organism by examination of a specimen of the discharge. It is very unwise to try to treat yourself by douching, since if you did happen to have something more serious than trichomonas, the flushing of infected material up into your womb or tubes could spread the infection and have tragic results.

My girlfriend has a trichomonas infection in her vagina. She says she hasn't been with anyone else, but since I have no symptoms and know that I have been only with her, is she deceiving me?

This is a situation that worries and upsets a lot of couples. However, the truth is, although it seems difficult to understand how a vaginal infection can be caught other than through intercourse with an infected person, a substantial proportion of cases are acquired not in this way, but by using a toilet that was contaminated by an infected person a short time before, or unwittingly borrowing an infected friend's towel or washcloth.

When I had trichomoniasis, my husband was given tablets even though there was nothing wrong with him. Why?

Though your husband may not have had trichomoniasis—it is not always sexually transmitted—he may have had a mild infection without any apparent symptoms. If this was the case you might have been reinfected when you started having intercourse after your treatment.

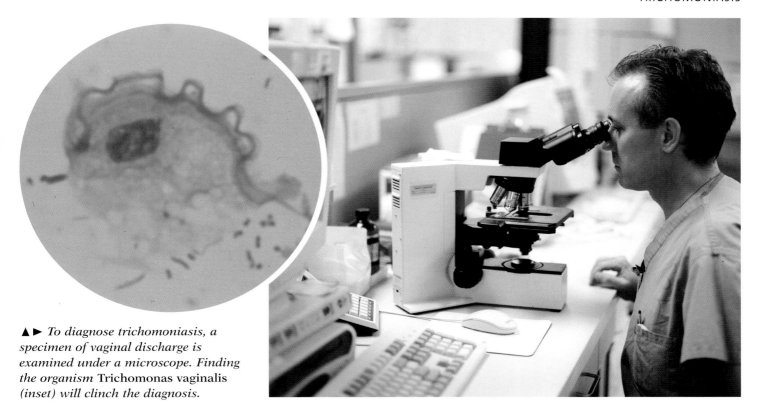

▲ ► *To diagnose trichomoniasis, a specimen of vaginal discharge is examined under a microscope. Finding the organism* Trichomonas vaginalis *(inset) will clinch the diagnosis.*

Although trichomoniasis can often be caught as a result of having intercourse with somebody who already has the infection, it can be contracted in other ways. Indeed, the fact that the trichomonas infection occurs in a much greater number of women than men, that it does not usually survive for long in males, and that the infection can develop in women who are not having intercourse confirms this. The answer to this apparent mystery lies in the ability of the trichomonas organism, unlike other sexually transmitted organisms such as the gonococcus, to survive outside the human body for at least 30 minutes on objects with which the genital parts of an infected person have come in contact.

Trichomoniasis is therefore one of the few sexually transmitted diseases that can in fact be caught from a toilet seat as well as from contaminated towels, washcloths, or clothes (see Sexually Transmitted Diseases).

Symptoms

Almost all cases of trichomoniasis can be easily and completely cured. Usually, its only manifestation is vaginitis (inflammation of the vagina), the main symptom of which is a profuse vaginal discharge. This is generally runny, is yellow to green in color, and has a strong odor. The discharge is often accompanied by soreness and irritation of the genital area. It is very unusual for any organ other than the vagina, either in the pelvis or elsewhere in the body, to be affected, and the infection has virtually no complications.

Diagnosis

The diagnosis of trichomoniasis can be made only by seeing the actual trichomonas organism under a microscope in a specimen of the vaginal discharge; there are no blood or other tests that will reveal it. There are a large number of diseases that can cause several different types of vaginal discharge. Even though the nature of the discharge strongly suggests trichomonas infection, this can be completely verified only by an internal examination and by microscopic analysis of the discharge. Since trichomoniasis can be cured completely by only one particular type of drug (there is no single treatment effective for all types of vaginal discharge), it is important that the trichomonas organism is positively identified. Vaginal examination and tests are particularly advisable if the infection may have been caught through casual sexual intercourse, since it is possible to have acquired other infections, such as gonorrhea or thrush, at the same time (see Gonorrhea; Thrush). It is wise, therefore, to confirm or eliminate the presence of other infections so that appropriate additional treatment can be given if necessary. A full investigation can be carried out at a treatment center or genitourinary clinic.

Treatment

The treatment of trichomonas infection usually consists of taking oral doses of metronidazole (Flagyl) or another closely related drug. It is important that the effectiveness of the cure is checked after treatment by the examination of vaginal secretion to make sure that no organism has survived. Until this has been done, the patient should refrain from intercourse to avoid the possibility of reinfection and of contaminating anyone else. Since a considerable proportion of cases are sexually transmitted, and to avoid a situation in which a couple will continually reinfect each other, the patient's partner is usually advised either to undergo the tests as well, or to take a course of metronidazole as a precaution. Oral metronidazole in the dosage necessary to cure trichomoniasis is unlikely to have significant side effects but some undesirable reactions have been seen with long-term treatment. The drug is, available, however, in the form of vaginal pessaries or vaginal gel.

See also: **Parasites; Sex**

Tropical diseases

Questions and Answers

I am planning a trip to India, and know that rabies is common there. Should I be vaccinated before I go?

There is now a safe and effective—though expensive—vaccine against rabies. Rabies is spread by animal bites. The risk to ordinary travelers is usually so small, however, that vaccination is not routinely advised before a vacation.

Last time I went to Tunisia I had a terrible attack of diarrhea that ruined my visit. Can I take anything with me next time to prevent this from happening again?

Your doctor may be able to give you some tablets to relieve the symptoms in case it should happen again. However, travelers' diarrhea is nearly always due to eating or drinking contaminated food or water, and strict hygiene is the best preventive measure. Diarrhea is nature's way of eliminating noxious agents from the body, so treatment should focus on replacing lost fluids and salts—this is of vital importance in hot climates. If diarrhea does not get better within a short time, contains blood or mucus, or is associated with fever, consult a doctor at once.

I'm planning a trip to South America, and am scared of poisonous snakes. Is there anything that I should take with me in case I get bitten?

Snakes bite in self-defense, so always wear boots when walking outdoors in snake-infested areas. Snakebites are very uncommon and, usually, little or no venom is injected, but it is still important to get to a hospital without delay. Dramatic measures such as cutting into bites or using tourniquets are unnecessary and can cause harm. Reassurance is the most important part of treatment. Antivenin can be dangerous, and should be administered only by medics.

The grim backdrop to most tropical diseases is the shocking conditions in which so many people live. Governments and medical teams are waging war against the havoc wreaked by these resilient enemies of humanity.

In spite of all the progress that has been made in modern medicine, large numbers of people around the world still die from tropical diseases. Although the medical profession now understands a great deal about how these diseases spread, and how they can be treated, they still maim, blind, disable, and cause suffering on a massive scale.

What are tropical diseases?

Tropical diseases include not only strange parasitic disorders like elephantiasis, but also rare and deadly fevers like Lassa fever or Marburg fever. Relatively few diseases occur only within the tropics. Diseases such as leprosy (now referred to as Hansen's disease) and plague, which most

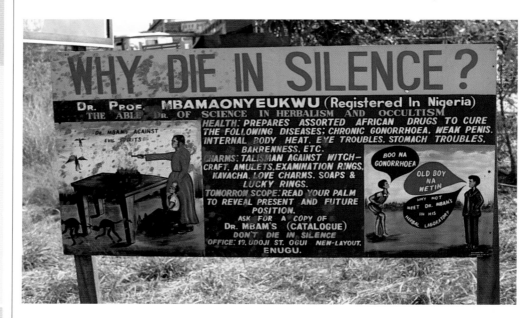

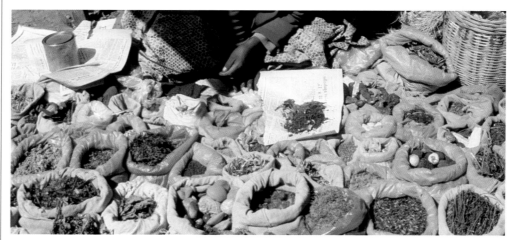

▲ *An African sign (top) promises bizarre cures for many complaints. A Peruvian herbalist displays his colorful herbal cure-alls for sale (above).*

people now think of as tropical, were once widespread in Europe (see Plague). Likewise, diseases now familiar in Europe, such as measles or tuberculosis, are much more dangerous in developing countries (see Measles). For example, the mortality from measles is 0.3 percent in European countries, compared to 1 to 10 percent in developing countries (see Infection and Infectious Diseases).

Fighting tropical diseases

Smallpox is the only disease totally eradicated by humans. The campaign against smallpox began in 1967, lasted 10 years, and cost $200 million (see Smallpox).

Although the World Health Organization (WHO) has a campaign to eradicate polio and leprosy from the world within a relatively short time, it is not likely that humankind will be able to eradicate many other tropical diseases in the foreseeable future, and much more money for research is necessary. However, the World Health Organization has determined that the following diseases should be singled out for particular attention.

Malaria: The disease affects an estimated 300 million people each year and causes over a million deaths. It is one of the world's greatest killers, and is still on the increase. Hopes of an effective vaccine against malaria have faded. Control depends largely on control of the insect that spreads it—the anopheles mosquito. Public health measures to remove mosquito breeding areas, and public knowledge of how the disease is spread, can help (see Public Health). New and more effective drugs to prevent and treat malaria are being developed.

Schistosomiasis: Also called bilharzia, this is an unpleasant and sometimes fatal disease caused by small worms in the liver,

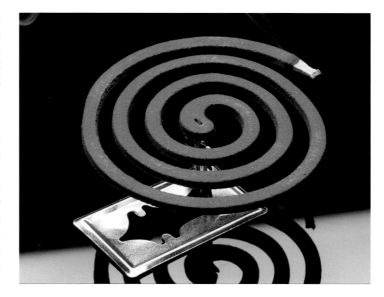

▲ *A pyrethrum mosquito coil should be burned at night to keep mosquitoes at bay in countries where malaria is rife.*

intestine, and bladder (see Worms). Eggs passed out in the urine and feces hatch in water and produce organisms that infect certain types of snails. These produce other types of organisms, which penetrate human skin and then pass in the bloodstream to the liver. The disease is usually caused by contact with water that has been contaminated by human sewage.

Sleeping sickness: Spread by the tsetse fly, this has made vast areas of Africa uninhabitable. The disease is caused by a tiny, single-celled parasite that lives in the

◀▼ *The spectacular wildlife of the Masai Mara game reserve attracts thousands of tourists to Kenya every year. However, such an area is home to the tsetse fly (below), which spreads sleeping sickness to both humans and animals. Mosquito coils should be standard travelers' equipment because they repel such unwanted visitors.*

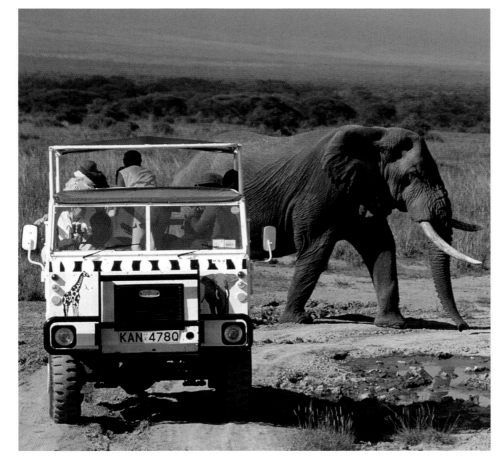

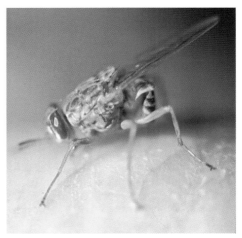

I've heard that cholera vaccination does not always work. Is there any other treatment for cholera?

A better vaccine is needed to fight cholera. At present, the vaccine protects in only 50 percent of cases for only a few months. Thus the best way to avoid cholera is to avoid food and water that might be contaminated. Cholera causes severe diarrhea, with salt and fluid loss. Prompt rehydration is vital in order to save a person's life.

My sister-in-law has just returned from a trip to Jamaica, where she became ill with dengue fever. What is dengue fever, and is there any chance that she could infect someone else?

Dengue is due to a virus. It is spread by certain types of mosquito, so you could not catch it directly from her. It causes fever, painful muscles and joints, headaches, and a rash, but complete recovery usually occurs.

Is it true that malnutrition can be caused by worms?

Intestinal parasites do not, on their own, cause malnutrition, although hookworms often cause anemia. However, in the tropics worm infestation in undernourished children is common, and often leads to severe malnutrition.

I am going to be touring the Middle East and I have heard that there is a disease there that causes blindness. Is there any chance that I might catch it?

The disease you are worried about is known as trachoma, an infection of the conjunctiva and cornea of the eye. Trachoma causes blindness on a massive scale: around 500 million people have the disease, of whom 15 million are now suffering from blindness. Repeated infection is necessary for damage to occur, and treatment with antibiotic ointment is highly effective. Travelers are most unlikely to be affected by it.

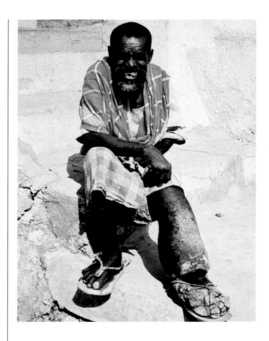

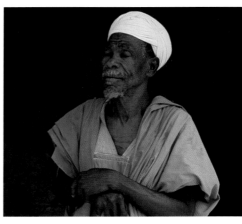

▲ *Blindness is a widespread tropical condition; in fact, one million people suffer from river blindness in West Africa alone.*

◄ *Elephantiasis is common in the tropics.*

blood and the brain, and causes serious damage to the nervous system (see Parasites). Treatment is difficult and there is no vaccine. The disease is a risk to visitors to African game parks, who should therefore take special precautions to avoid insect bites (see Bites and Stings).

Hansen's disease: This still affects a large number of people around the world. There are probably 20 million sufferers, though no more than 3 million receive treatment. If the disease is

Basic precautions

At present, many tropical diseases cannot be prevented by drugs or vaccines, so travelers should take a few basic precautions:

Biting insects spread diseases in different countries. In some parts of Africa, tsetse flies spread sleeping sickness; in others, insects spread viral diseases or filariasis. Minimize exposure to biting insects, and wear sensible clothes. Use insect repellents containing diethyltoluamide (DEET), and at night use a mosquito net or burn pyrethrum mosquito coils. Electronic insect repellents do not work.

Don't eat food that has been exposed to flies. Always eat food that has been freshly cooked to kill all parasites and bacteria. Wash hands before handling food.

Check that drinking water is safe; if in doubt, drink boiled water, or use purifying tablets containing chlorine or iodine.

Wash fruit and vegetables with detergent or a dilute solution of potassium permanganate.

Never walk around barefoot.

Cleanse and dress all wounds.

Do not swim in canals or rivers.

If you develop a fever, severe diarrhea, or blood in the feces, consult a doctor.

Have a medical checkup when you return home.

diagnosed promptly, it can be treated effectively and disability can be prevented. However, if it is neglected, blindness, paralysis, and deformity result. Almost more terrible is the social stigma of the disease due to the ancient and irrational fear of infection. This causes the sufferer to become a social outcast. More effective drugs are badly needed, as well as vaccine research.

Filariasis: This disease is caused by a variety of small worms that enter the body through the bites of mosquitoes and flies. These worms also cause elephantiasis by blocking the lymph passages in the body. African river blindness is another form of filariasis. This can cause blindness by infestation with a worm that enters the body through a blackfly bite. There are over 250 million cases of filariasis.

Leishmaniasis: Spread by sandflies, and caused by a parasite that attacks the skin, liver, and spleen, the disease takes many forms and is not adequately understood. More research is needed.

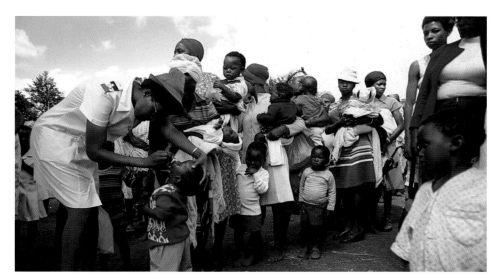

▲ *Massive vaccination programs are taking place in Africa.*

high dam controlled the floods of the Nile and permitted much better irrigation and crop yields. Although this was a benefit, it also, however, allowed the snails that transmit bilharzia to flourish. It is

Immunization schemes

Measles, diphtheria, polio, tetanus, tuberculosis, and whooping cough (medically known as pertussis) kill five million children in developing countries each year (see Diphtheria). The World Health Organization set itself a huge task: to immunize all children in the world against these diseases by the year 2000 (see Immunization). The target was not met, but good progress was made. The practical problems are enormous, since 80 percent of the world's population live in remote areas. Even when supplies of vaccine arrive, their effectiveness cannot always be guaranteed; vaccines are quickly inactivated by tropical heat.

Problems

Poverty, overpopulation, overcrowding, bad housing, inadequate nutrition, poor sanitation, and lack of education are a few of the factors that facilitate the spread of tropical diseases in the developing world, and make them more difficult to bring under control (see Hygiene; Malnutrition). A billion people have no access to a safe water supply within 220 yards (200 m) of their home.

Ironically, many aid projects aimed at improving the quality of life have actually made things worse. In Egypt, for example, the construction of the Aswān

Facts about malaria
Malaria is one of the leading causes of sickness and death in the developing world.
About 35 percent of the world's population—about two billion people—are at risk.
At least 80 percent of deaths from malaria occur in sub-Saharan Africa, where the disease kills at least one million people each year.
According to the World Health Organization, there are 300 million to 500 million new clinical cases of malaria every year.
In 2001, malaria resulted in an estimated 1.5 million to 2.7 million deaths.
Children aged one to four are the most vulnerable to infection and death.
Malaria causes as many as half the deaths of African children under the age of five.
The disease kills more than one million children each year in Africa alone.
In some regions of high incidence, 40 percent of toddlers may die of acute malaria.
Malaria is now spreading to areas previously free of the disease.
Mosquitoes are developing resistance to pesticides.
Malarial parasites are developing resistance to treatment drugs.
The Centers for Disease Control received reports of 1,383 cases of malaria in the United States in 2001. Only two of these cases were acquired in the United States.

Why do babies who are suffering from malnutrition have such enormous abdomens when the rest of their bodies seem to be just skin and bones?

The swollen abdomen of the malnourished child is due to wasting and weakening of the abdominal muscles, fluid collecting in the abdomen, gas distending the intestines, and an enlarged liver. This type of malnutrition, called kwashiorkor, results from a diet containing little or no protein, and carries a high mortality rate.

Is it true that there is resistance to various antimalarial drugs among certain malaria strains, rendering these drugs ineffective?

In some parts of Africa, Asia, and South America, resistance to some of the drugs used to prevent malaria is now increasing. Check with your doctor before you travel, explaining exactly which countries you plan to visit, so that he or she can select the most suitable treatment. Don't forget that even the shortest stopover in a tropical zone may expose you to malaria.

Is vaccination against certain tropical diseases dangerous during pregnancy?

If there is a significant risk of exposure to disease, vaccination is usually the safest option. Ask your doctor for his or her advise.

I thought that leprosy was found only in underdeveloped countries, but I read recently that it still occurs in Europe and the United States. Is this true?

It is true, but it is nothing for you to worry about. Leprosy (Hansen's disease) has never been eradicated completely from Europe or the United States. There are probably about 20 million sufferers from the disease in the world. However, contrary to commonly held beliefs, Hansen's disease does not spread easily, and most people are not at all susceptible to the disease.

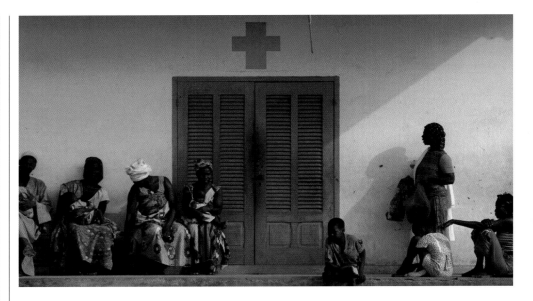

▲ *Women and children from an Ivory Coast village await treatment in the local community hospital.*

estimated that 60 percent of Egypt's population suffers from bilharzia, and that 200 million people in Southeast Asia, Africa, and South America are affected.

The countries in which tropical diseases are most common are those least able to conduct the intensive research that is essential if new drugs and vaccines to combat these diseases are to be found. They simply do not have the financial and technological resources.

It costs many millions of dollars to research and test each new drug, and developing countries can barely afford the drugs that are already available.

Travel

Jet travel has made it possible for a disease acquired in one country to produce symptoms only after the traveler has arrived in another country, often many thousands of miles away. Yellow

▼ *Attempts to control the spread of river blindness have included the introduction of public showers in India.*

▼ *With the help of better health education and medical care, African children have real hope of a longer, healthier life.*

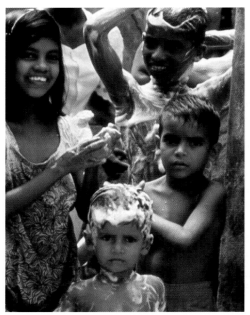

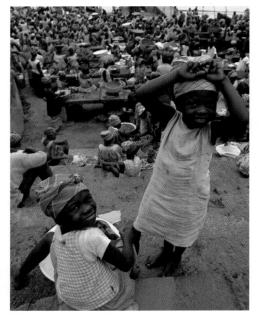

Travel precautions

If you are planning to visit a country where tropical diseases are present, see your doctor well in advance to allow plenty of time for any immunizations you may need. You will probably require specific protection against the diseases listed below.

DISEASE	PROTECTIVE MEASURES	DOSAGE	DURATION OF PROTECTION	EFFECTS OF DISEASE	ROUTE OF DISEASE SPREAD
Cholera	Immunization Hygiene	2 doses, 1–4 weeks apart	6 months	Severe diarrhea, fluid loss, and dehydration	Unhygienic food handling, and contaminated water
Hepatitis	Gammaglobulin injection Vaccine for hepatitis B	Single dose 3 doses	2–6 months Life	Fever, jaundice, viral liver infection	Contact with infected cases, unhygienic food handling, contaminated water
Malaria	Antimalarial drugs Mosquito nets Mosquito repellents	Start drug treatment before arrival, continue for at least 6 weeks after leaving	During period of exposure	Fevers and chills	Mosquito bites
Polio	Oral polio vaccine Hygiene	Single booster dose, if previously immunized	5 years	Paralysis	Unhygienic food handling, and contaminated water
Smallpox	Vaccination is no longer required or advised. The disease has been eradicated.				
Tetanus	Immunization. Careful cleansing of cuts and wounds.	2 doses, 4–6 weeks apart. 1st booster dose 1 year later; then every 5 years	5–10 years	Severe muscle spasms and rigidity	Contamination of a wound or wounds
Tuberculosis	BCG immunization (following skin test)	Single dose	Probably lifelong	Chronic lung disease; damage to many organs	Direct contact with infected cases; unpasteurized milk
Typhoid	Immunization Hygiene	2 doses, 4 weeks apart	3 years	Fever; intestinal infection	Unhygienic food handling, and contaminated water
Yellow fever	Immunization	Single dose	10 years	Fever, also jaundice, bleeding	Mosquito bites

fever, for example, which is a dangerous viral illness (see Viruses) occurring in Africa and South America, is transmitted by mosquitoes, and the symptoms do not appear until six days after a mosquito bite. International health regulations ensure that all travelers arriving in Asia from Africa or South America have been vaccinated against yellow fever for their own safety, and to prevent the spread of the disease. There is, at present, no yellow fever in Asia, although there are plenty of mosquitoes that would be able to spread the disease rapidly.

Only a few tropical diseases can be prevented specifically by drug treatment or by vaccination, so travelers to regions where diseases are endemic must accept that they are at an increased risk of picking up a disease against which they have no natural immunity.

An additional hazard is that when particular symptoms develop after a traveler has returned home, they may not be recognized immediately as symptoms of a tropical disease. In the West, over 2,500 cases of malaria are imported each year, but the symptoms are easily confused with those of influenza and the diagnosis is often delayed. Travelers should, therefore, always tell their doctor where they have been when they return home, and should have a full checkup.

Outlook

Many tropical diseases are on the increase, and are a long way from eradication or control. Improved health education and public health services are the most urgent measures that must be taken to limit the spread of tropical diseases. New vaccines, new drugs, and more research are essential if the fight against tropical diseases is to succeed.

See also: **Cholera; Elephantiasis; Hansen's disease; Hookworms; Malaria; Poliomyelitis; Travel and health; Tuberculosis; Vaccinations; Yellow fever**

Tubal ligation

Questions and Answers

I want to be sterilized. If I have tubal ligation, will I be able to have the procedure reversed if I decide that I want another baby?

Female or male sterilization should be considered only if you are sure that you will never want another child. It offers a virtually 100 percent safe form of birth control, and must be regarded as an irreversible procedure. In certain circumstances surgeons may try to reverse the procedure, but there is no guarantee that they will be successful. In women, the success rate of the reversal procedure is only around 50 percent, and the pregnancy rate in the partners of men who have had vasectomies reversed is no more than 60 percent.

Does a woman who has had tubal ligation go through menopause after she has had this surgery?

No. The procedure simply involves tying each of the fallopian tubes in two places and destroying the section in between to prevent sperm from reaching the eggs. The ovaries are not affected and continue to produce both eggs and sex hormones. However, some female sterilization procedures involve removing or damaging the ovaries, and afterward, a woman will develop menopausal symptoms, such as hot flashes. Such a method is carried out only if the ovaries are already damaged or diseased.

My wife is having tubal ligation. Will we have to use any other contraception after surgery?

No. Female sterilization is effective immediately, so no form of contraception is necessary. After a vasectomy it is possible for a man to remain fertile for three months, and couples should use a form of contraception until a sample of semen shows no sperm.

Tubal ligation is a simple sterilization procedure that is performed on a woman's fallopian tubes to prevent sperm from reaching the eggs, or on a man's vas deferens to prevent the passage of sperm from the testes.

The word "ligation" means tying off or constriction. In tubal ligation, it is the tubes that carry the eggs in a woman or the sperm in a man that are tied, and this makes a woman or man unable to reproduce—a procedure called sterilization (see Sterilization; Vasectomy).

Men or women who have completed their families or who do not want children may be sterilized so that they do not have to worry about contraception or unwanted pregnancies. Tubal ligation may be considered if a pregnancy would be a serious threat to a woman's health, or if there is a high risk that children would be affected by a serious hereditary disease.

How is it done?

Tubal ligation in women is carried out by keyhole surgery through a small incision in the abdomen and is performed under local or spinal anesthesia. Each fallopian tube is tied in two places by a tight ligature, and the segment between is removed. Sometimes a loop of the tube is tied with a tight band, but the tube is not cut so that, in theory, the sterilization procedure can be reversed. Although this procedure is more commonly carried out through a small incision in the abdomen, the procedure can be performed vaginally under local anesthesia.

The procedure in men, known as vasectomy, can be carried out at a day clinic under local anesthesia. The surgeon makes two small incisions in the scrotum (see Penis and Disorders), cuts each of the two vasa deferentia (the extensions of the testis that run from the scrotum to join the seminal vesicle that forms the ejaculatory duct), and ties the cut ends. This procedure makes a man sterile by interrupting the route of the spermatozoa.

Both women and men will experience some tenderness after such sterilization surgery, but any pain can be controlled with nonprescription painkillers. After the procedure a woman becomes infertile because sperm cannot reach the egg. However, a man remains fertile after a vasectomy until any sperm already present in each vas deferens have been ejaculated or die. For this reason, alternative contraception must be used until the man has produced two consecutive sperm-free specimens.

▲ *In female sterilization, the vagina is clamped open and an incision is made near the cervix (at center). The fallopian tubes are drawn through the vaginal wall and ligatured, and are then pushed back into the abdominal cavity. The incision is then stitched up.*

Success rate

The failure rate of the sterilization procedure in women is about one in 1,000, and if a woman becomes pregnant afterward (a very rare occurrence), there is an increased risk of an ectopic pregnancy (see Ectopic Pregnancy).

In men, the two ends of a severed vas deferens may join up again over a period of time, but this occurs very rarely.

Under exceptional circumstances a surgeon may try to reverse the sterilization procedure in a man or in a woman who has not had the fallopian tubes cut, just looped. In such cases, the success rate of reversal in both sexes is about 50 percent.

See also: **Minimally invasive surgery**

Tuberculosis

Questions and Answers

Can I get TB from milk?

Two strains of the TB bacterium are important causes of the disease in humans. The first is the human strain, and the second is the bovine strain that can be passed on in milk. However, because cattle are now tested for infection—so-called tuberculin-tested herds—the bovine strain is no longer passed on in milk.

My grandfather had several ribs cut away because of TB, and was left with a deformed chest. Why?

Before antibiotics became available, surgery was one of the few ways of fighting TB. One method was to cut out the affected parts of the lung, although this was a major operation, and the disease was likely to affect both lungs. Another approach was to reduce the volume of areas of affected lung, since the disease caused cavities, particularly in the upper parts of the lung. If the cavities were removed there seemed to be a better chance of curing the disease. This sort of surgery is no longer necessary, since drugs can now cure the disease.

Can I be vaccinated against tuberculosis?

Yes you can. There is a vaccine called BCG, which is a modified form of the TB bacterium. This can fire the immune system against the disease but does not cause serious disease. Children at special risk are tested for evidence of previous contact with the disease (primary TB) and, if they are negative to testing, they are given BCG. Children who react are known as tuberculin-positive and are immune. People at risk from the disease, such as medics, are tested and revaccinated as necessary. Mass vaccination is not carried out in the United States.

Thanks to improved nutrition and living conditions, tuberculosis is no longer prevalent in the developed West, although in recent years there has been a resurgence of a resistant form of the disease in inner-city areas.

Tuberculosis—or TB as it is more commonly known—remains one of the most serious infectious diseases in the world. Although improved standards of living conditions have made the disease less prevalent in the West, it remains a killer in the developing world.

TB is caused by a funguslike bacterium called *Mycobacterium tuberculosis*, and there are two main strains of this particular organism that cause disease in humans; a human strain and a bovine strain, which primarily infects cattle, but which is also capable of causing human disease (see Bacteria). The incidence of this chronic infection and the problems it can cause vary from country to country. In the United States, infection of the lungs—pulmonary TB—is the most usual form of the disease, whereas in Africa abdominal TB is very common.

How TB develops

At one time most people growing up in a country like the United States would have been in contact with tuberculosis at an early age. Such early contact with the disease leads to an infection called primary TB, which often, but not always, has no significant symptoms. The disease is contracted by contact with someone who has sufficiently severe disease in the lungs to cough up sputum containing TB bacteria. If the amount of bacteria inhaled is relatively small, then the primary TB will be a minor infection that will help build up a partial immunity to the development of full-blown TB later on (see Immune System).

The more serious forms of the disease that occur in later life are called postprimary disease. It seems that the usual cause of these infections is that the immunity to the original infection has broken down and the TB bacteria have literally broken out of their original site. Although this is probably the usual mechanism of development of the disease, it is also likely that some people who develop TB later in life do so because they are exposed to a very high infecting dose of bacteria. The reasons immunity breaks down are not clear. In most cases it seems that social rather than medical factors are of significance, since there is little doubt that TB these days is a disease most common among vagrants and alcoholics, although it may still occur in an apparently fit person who is well fed and lives in good housing. Because of the loss of immunity, the World Health Organization (WHO) estimates that one-third of people who are HIV-positive are infected with *M. tuberculosis* and will develop overt TB. TB rates in the United States, which had been falling steadily, showed a rise again around 1987, largely because of AIDS but also because of growing social deprivation.

Complications of primary TB

Although primary TB is often a relatively minor infection with no symptoms, it can develop into a serious disease in young children or in children who have another debilitating disease. The site of infection is nearly always the lungs, although in some parts of the world it may be the abdomen. The original infection causes a small area of

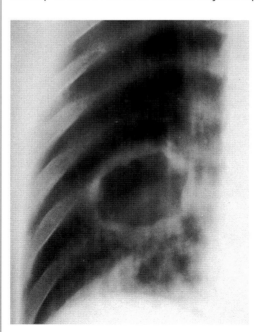

▲ *This X ray of a lung shows a large cavity created by a primary TB infection; bacilli are still contained inside it.*

Questions and Answers

Is it true that you have to be hospitalized for months to be cured of TB?

No. If you are found to have TB these days, you won't necessarily have to be in the hospital at all. In the past there was no effective cure, and it was found that rest in a sanitarium was beneficial. People who could afford it were sent away to mountain resorts where the purer air was thought to be helpful. Today the drug treatment is so efficient that you are no longer infectious after about 10 days. However, the standard length of treatment for pulmonary TB is still nine months.

My friend had TB which affected the liver and abdomen. Isn't TB usually a chest disease?

You are right in thinking that the disease normally affects the chest. However, disease outside the chest does occur, although it is not very common in the United States. One of the most interesting things about TB is the way it presents itself in different ways in different groups of people. Immigrants to the United States from Africa or India are much more likely to have TB in areas other than the chest than someone who was born here. This does not seem to be due to racial differences, since the children of immigrant parents who are born and raised in this country seem to get TB in the lungs if they do happen to develop it.

Is it true that modern drugs are so effective that TB is no longer a common problem?

It is true that the disease is much less common than it used to be, and that the drugs to treat the disease are very effective. However, there is little evidence that the two facts are related. TB was on the decline before the drugs were widely available. It is thought that the combination of improved housing and improved nutrition is the main reason for the reduced incidence of TB.

inflammation in one of the lungs, and this produces a reaction in the lymph nodes that drain lymphatic fluids from that part of the lung. This patch of inflammation and enlargement of some of the lymph nodes at the root of the lung is called the primary complex.

In most cases, the TB bacteria in the primary complex are contained by the lymph nodes and spread no farther, but in a few children and adolescents with primary TB the defense mechanism breaks down soon after infection. This allows the bacteria to spread throughout the body, leading to a serious condition called miliary TB, which causes general illness, with loss of weight and a high fever. Diagnosis is by X-ray examination of the chest, which shows that both lungs are full of tiny nodules, each of which represents an area of tuberculous infection. Sometimes the general spread of the disease soon after the primary infection leads to an infection in the

PROGRESS OF PULMONARY TUBERCULOSIS

Advanced TB usually results when a dormant primary infection is reactivated and the bacteria spread to cause extensive cavitation in both lungs (below). The blood vessels then become congested and are likely to rupture, causing hemorrhage.

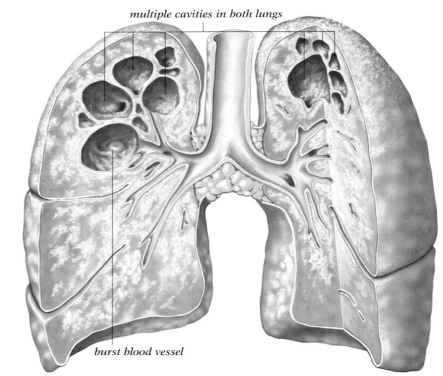

multiple cavities in both lungs

burst blood vessel

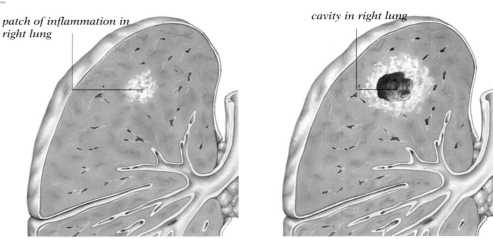

patch of inflammation in right lung

cavity in right lung

▲ *TB begins as a small inflamed area in one lung (above left), which turns into a cavity (above right).*

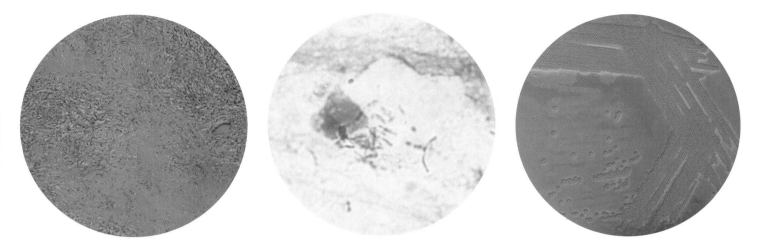

▲ *Untreated TB can lead to infection of the pleura (the membranes encasing the lungs) and then to pleural fibrosis (above left). This is usually very rigid, being full of calcium, and will impede breathing. When stained, any bacteria will appear as thin red rods (above center). If the diagnosis is unclear, a bacterial culture is grown on a plate (above right).*

nervous system called TB meningitis. Unlike the more common types of meningitis that develop within a day or so of infection, TB meningitis may take some weeks to develop (see Meningitis). The first symptoms are general ill health, a slight fever, headaches (a very unusual complaint in a child), and, occasionally, fits. At a later stage, the fever rises and signs of drowsiness and neck stiffness appear. Finally, the temperature rises even higher and obvious problems with individual nerves, such as those controlling the eyes, will occur. This is a very dangerous condition, and it is important to start treatment as soon as the diagnosis is made. The diagnosis is confirmed by performing a lumbar puncture, which enables doctors to examine the cerebrospinal fluid that bathes the brain and spinal cord (see Lumbar Puncture). One of the findings that indicate TB meningitis is a level of sugar in the fluid that is very much lower than that in the blood. This finding is almost unique to this particular condition.

Pulmonary TB

Although the primary focus of pulmonary TB occurs in the lungs, it is not until the postprimary stage of infection that there are any problems in the lungs. In a few cases of primary TB, the lymph nodes at the root of the lung may break down and liberate the bacteria into one of the main tubes (bronchi) supplying a particular lobe of the lung. This in turn will lead to lobar pneumonia soon after the original infection.

Most cases of tuberculous lung disease, however, happen many years after the original infection with the disease. The primary focus has a tendency to attack the lower lobes of the lungs, whereas the postprimary infection is much more likely to occur in the highest segments of the upper lobes of the lungs. It seems that the large amounts of oxygen that are available there, together with the relatively poor supply of blood, create particularly suitable incubators for the lung disease.

When the disease has become established in the upper part of the lungs, it may cause cavities to form there. Once this has happened, large numbers of TB bacteria may be present in the sputum, and this means that the sufferer becomes a serious source of infection until he or she is treated. The sufferer is most likely to infect young children, giving them primary TB, TB meningitis, or TB bronchopneumonia. It is even possible that someone spreading large numbers of TB bacteria is able to rekindle the disease in people in older age groups who have already suffered from the primary form of the illness.

Left untreated, pulmonary TB can lead to the formation of fluid in the pleural space that surrounds the lungs, to infection of the pleura (lining membrane), and subsequently to pleural thickening and fibrosis (see Pleurisy). A particular characteristic of TB is that the fibrosis it leaves behind is often full of calcium and is therefore very rigid. Obviously, a lung surrounded by a hard wrapping of bonelike fibrosis is not going to be able to move freely, and breathing will be seriously impaired.

Sometimes the same sequence of events will happen to the pericardium—the membranous sac that surrounds the heart. This has even more serious effects, since tuberculous pericarditis may restrict the activity of the heart and stop it from pumping enough blood to the rest of the body.

Diagnosis

It is usually easy to diagnose a case of pulmonary TB. In a well-developed infection there will be marked changes on the chest X ray, particularly in the upper parts of the two upper lobes. One of the difficulties in diagnosing from an X ray, however, is identifying whether the changes represent a new infection of tuberculosis or an old infection. The fibrosis caused by an early episode of TB will persist for life, and the changes in the lungs will be visible on any chest X-ray for the remainder of the patient's life.

In a case of suspected tuberculosis, the first laboratory test will be to inspect the patient's sputum under a microscope. When there is a heavy infection, the sputum will contain a lot of bacteria. These will show up as thin red rods when stained with a special stain called Ziehl-Neelsen stain. The presence or absence of bacteria on direct staining of the sputum is of great relevance, since if there are no bacteria the patient cannot be infectious, even if he or she does turn out to have TB at a later stage. Infection with the presence of bacteria on direct staining is called open TB, and this is the only type that can possibly be infectious.

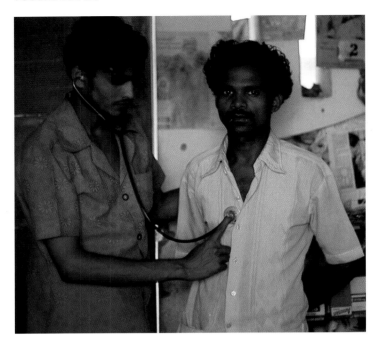

▲ *TB is a pervasive problem in India, but there are now clinics set up where people can be diagnosed and treated.*

Other forms of TB

Although pulmonary TB is the most common form of the disease, there are many other areas of the body that it may attack, such as the uterus, genitals, kidney, skin, and spine.

Abdominal tuberculosis

Abdominal TB is a common problem, particularly in Africa and India. It can be difficult to make a confident diagnosis, since there is no convenient test, such as a chest X ray, that confirms the disease. Sufferers simply appear to be generally rather sick, and will have a raised temperature. A simple way to make a diagnosis is by performing a liver biopsy: that is, surgically removing a small piece of liver and examining it under a microscope to see if any TB bacteria are present (see Biopsy).

TB may also attack the lymph glands in the neck, and cause an abscess to form (see Abscess), which sometimes involves the overlying skin. This condition is called scrofula.

Treatment

Prior to the 1950s, when there was no effective drug treatment available, TB was often fatal. The cure for pulmonary TB, for instance, relied on building up the patient's resistance with rest and nourishment. However, this care often came too late. The clarity of the air and the relative lack of oxygen at great heights were also thought to be helpful, and there were many sanitariums in mountain resorts where wealthy TB sufferers went to recover.

Surgery was also routinely performed to remove severely infected areas of the lungs. This reduced the volume of the lungs and obliterated the cavities, thereby halting the spread of the disease through the lungs.

However, before antibiotics were introduced as a treatment for TB (see Antibiotics), attempts to achieve a cure were frustrated by the fact that the disease was often widespread before treatment was started. This often resulted in very intense fibrous scarring of the lung tissue, which prevented it from fulfilling the function of transferring oxygen from the air into the blood. Even today, if cases of TB are left untreated for too long, fibrosis will occur and this condition cannot be helped by antibiotics.

With modern treatment, however, it is possible to stop the progress of TB within a few days of starting treatment, although it can take as many as nine months to achieve a complete cure. There are now a selection of drugs that can be used to treat the TB infection. The first of these was streptomycin and, although still used, it is somewhat limited by the fact that it has to be given by injection. The usual drugs used today include rifampin, rifabutin, isoniazid, and ethambutol.

To prevent the organism from becoming resistant to any one drug, it is customary to use a combination of drugs during the early stages of the infection. Once the organism has grown—and this may take three months—it is possible to show that it is sensitive to at least two of the drugs and one is then withdrawn. The length of time it takes to cure TB varies depending on the particular type of infection: at least nine months in the case of pulmonary TB, but much longer in the case of abdominal TB.

Prevention

It is possible to test the population for immunity to TB using a preparation of TB-derived protein called tuberculin. People with a partial immunity to the disease as a result of a primary TB infection in the past will show a reaction when tuberculin is injected into the skin. In cases of established postprimary TB the extent of the reaction will be greater. If a child between the ages of 11 and 13 has not yet come into contact with the disease, then it is well worth vaccinating him or her with BCG (bacille Calmette-Guérin), a vaccine that is a modified form of the TB bacterium. The vaccine produces the same effect as a minor primary infection, and gives a certain amount of immunity against the disease. It is also worthwhile having younger children vaccinated when there is a risk of contact with the disease.

However, the most effective prevention is to improve risk factors such as living conditions and poor diet. This advancement has reduced the incidence of TB in countries like the United States. Although the introduction of curative drugs was undoubtedly important, the number of people suffering from the disease had actually started to decline before these drugs became available. Today, TB is very uncommon in well-nourished, well-housed communities, and it is likely that TB would disappear altogether if everyone lived under such conditions.

Reported cases of tuberculosis in United States	
Data estimated by the Centers for Disease Control and Prevention	
YEAR	CASES
1980	28,000
1985	22,000
1990	26,000
1995	23,000
1996	21,000
1997	20,000
1998	18,000
1999	17,500
2000	15,500
2001	14,000
2002	12,000

See also: Infection and infectious diseases; Lymphatic system; Vaccinations

Tumors

It can be very alarming to discover a growth or swelling, which a doctor would describe as a tumor. In fact, some tumors are harmless or benign, and many others respond to treatment—especially if they are diagnosed early.

Questions and Answers

What is the difference between a cancer and a tumor?

The term "cancer" is used to describe any malignant tumor. The medical terms for cancer are "carcinoma" and "sarcoma." A carcinoma is a tumor arising from a lining membrane, whereas a sarcoma arises in connective tissue, like fat or muscle. When doctors use the words "growth" or "tumor" they could mean one that is benign or malignant.

My doctor thinks I may have an abdominal tumor, and has referred me to a surgeon at the hospital. What will happen next?

The surgeon will examine your abdomen to help locate the tumor. He or she will then arrange for you to have some scans or X rays to support the diagnosis. Any subsequent treatment will depend on the type of tumor and its location.

My father had a tumor removed from his colon. Could it recur?

Yes, the surgeon will have some information about the tumor's spread after surgery. There may also be evidence of any secondary tumors from X rays and other tests. The surgeon will have examined a piece of tissue from the tumor under the microscope, and this will tell him or her more about the growth's malignancy.

Do malignant tumors develop quickly, and are they always fatal?

By no means. Some malignant tumors are so slow-growing that they are unlikely to spread at all. Many other tumors can be treated very successfully with surgery, radiotherapy, or a course of chemotherapy. To a large extent, successful treatment depends on early diagnosis.

Any type of abnormal growth should be called a tumor. This can cause distressing misunderstandings, since medical personnel tend to use the term accurately, whereas laypeople often mistakenly think that all tumors are malignant or cancerous growths.

The body's normal cells are subject to controls that ensure that new cells are made at the same rate at which the old cells are lost. For example, as skin cells are destroyed by friction and abrasion on the surface, equal numbers of new cells form. Therefore, the skin is roughly the same thickness throughout life. The exact mechanics of this control system are not understood, but if it breaks down, cells are formed at an unchecked rate and a tumor is formed.

Types of tumor

There are two basic types of tumor; benign and malignant. Benign tumors are localized growths of tissue that produce swellings. There is no tendency for these extra cells to spread or grow into other parts of the body. However, these tumors can have serious consequences as a result of their location. For example, a benign tumor of the nerve tissue in the spinal canal can put pressure on the spinal cord, causing paralysis (see Paralysis). Similarly, an organ may be damaged if pressure is put on one of the blood vessels that supply it. The major identifying characteristic of malignant tumors is that they have a tendency to spread to other parts of the body. However, it can still be extremely difficult to diagnose a tumor as malignant, since some tumors are, in fact, very slow-growing. Malignant tumors are separated into two further groups; primary and secondary. The original tumor is known as the primary one. As this grows, fragments of the tissue may break off and settle in other parts of the body. These then multiply and the cells that make up the fragments form secondary tumors. Secondary tumor cells can usually be identified under a microscope because they consist of cells that are normally found in another part of the body. For instance, a primary tumor of the thyroid gland may spread to the bones, so that a secondary tumor formed of abnormal thyroid cells is found in a bone.

How malignant tumors spread

Malignant tumors can spread in many ways: through blood vessels or lymphatic channels, by direct extension into organs, or by growing across body cavities.

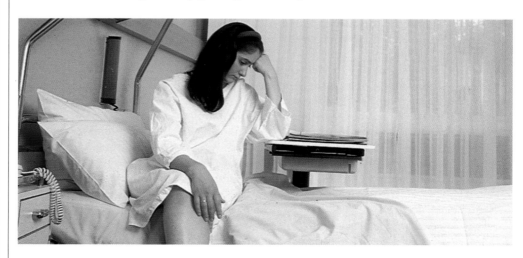

▲ *A patient who is waiting for the diagnosis of a tumor will be understandably apprehensive and anxious about the future.*

HOW TUMORS SPREAD

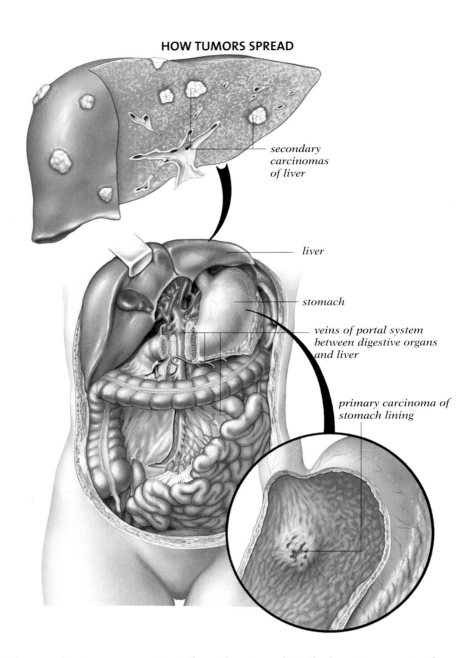

secondary
carcinomas
of liver

liver

stomach

veins of portal system
between digestive organs
and liver

primary carcinoma of
stomach lining

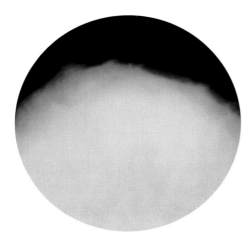

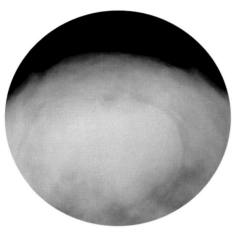

▲ *A mammograph, a type of X ray, is used to diagnose breast tumors. The right breast is normal (top) while the left shows a tumor (above).*

Small clumps of cells can break off from a primary tumor and enter the veins that drain the tissue around the tumor. The fragments are carried back to the heart and on to the lungs, where the cells can lodge and grow.

Cancer can spread through blood vessels or lymph vessels. The body has a system of tiny channels that carry lymph to and from the lymph glands. Tumor cells can enter this system and cause secondary tumors in the lymph glands. The secondaries are sometimes quite some distance from the primary tumor. For example, a tumor in one of the testes can sometimes lead to a secondary tumor in the neck.

Tumors can also spread when affected cells extend into adjacent tissues. This can make treatment particularly difficult, since completely removing the tumor may involve cutting away a vital part of a neighboring organ.

Finally, tumors can spread across spaces in the body such as the abdominal or chest cavities. A malignant stomach tumor may sometimes spread across the peritoneum (the membrane that lines the abdomen) so that secondaries occur in the pelvis (see Abdomen; Pelvis; Peritoneum).

▲ *The portal veins carry nutrients from the stomach to the liver. Fragments of a malignant tumor may be transported to the liver and secondaries may grow there.*

Treatment

The treatment for tumors varies enormously. Benign tumors are usually removed, unless their location makes them unlikely to cause problems. Malignant tumors can be treated by surgical removal, radiotherapy, or chemotherapy. Surgery is the preferred treatment, but sometimes it is not possible to operate; for example, the patient may not be strong enough to undergo surgery. Radiotherapy and chemotherapy (see Cancer; Radiotherapy) both destroy the rapidly dividing cells that are found in malignant tumors.

Each type of treatment for tumors has side effects, particularly chemotherapy, which can also damage normal body cells. However, the benefits of these treatments can vastly outweigh these effects.

See also: **Mammography; Side effects; Surgery; X rays**

Twitches and tics

Questions and Answers

When I am tired I get a twitching in the corner of my eye. Is there anything wrong?

No. This happens to people when they are tired or irritated, and it is quite normal. Occasionally, such a twitch may become ingrained and happen more frequently; it is then called a tic.

My young daughter has started grimacing for no reason. Is it a tic, and what can be done about it?

This may well be a tic. Tics are frequent in the five- to ten-year-old age group. If the matter is not made into a major issue and your daughter is not made aware of it, the tic will probably disappear. Other tics may show themselves from time to time, but they need not cause concern.

Sometimes, just as I am going to sleep, I get powerful twitching in my arms and legs. What is it?

This is known as a myoclonic jerk, and it is not unusual in the early stages of sleep. It is harmless, and there is nothing to worry about. It is, in fact, one of the most common forms of twitches, and can be so violent that it shakes the person back to consciousness.

My son has a mild form of epilepsy and recently, in addition to his occasional seizures, he sometimes has sudden twitching of his muscles, particularly when he is using them. Does this mean his epilepsy is getting worse?

Probably not. This is another form of myoclonus and is a common feature of epilepsy, especially in children. It can be associated with serious brain damage, but is usually just a symptom of the electrical instability of the brain as well as your son's tendency to have epileptic seizures.

Most people prefer to have control of the actions of their body, and would find it alarming if they found themselves making lots of involuntary movements. However, most of these movements are simply twitches or tics.

Occasional twitches of our muscles happen to all of us from time to time, but in some disorders of the nervous system these involuntary movements may become numerous and troublesome. Sometimes a repeated twitch in a particular group of muscles, particularly in the face, may take on a stereotyped pattern, and it is then referred to as a tic. Larger-scale jumps of the muscle, called myoclonic jerks, are also common.

What causes twitching?

When operating normally, muscles contract smoothly and evenly, and work together to produce coordinated movements (see Muscles). However, a twitch in a group of muscles happens in isolation and obviously does not result in any planned action. The body has a complex movement control system designed to eliminate such wasteful actions, so a twitch usually indicates some minor breakdown in the system.

The most common time for motor control to be upset and a twitch to occur is when we are tired (see Tiredness). It is usual for the odd twitch to occur around the eyelids, for example, when we are feeling drowsy. More severe disturbances can occur when the metabolic systems of the

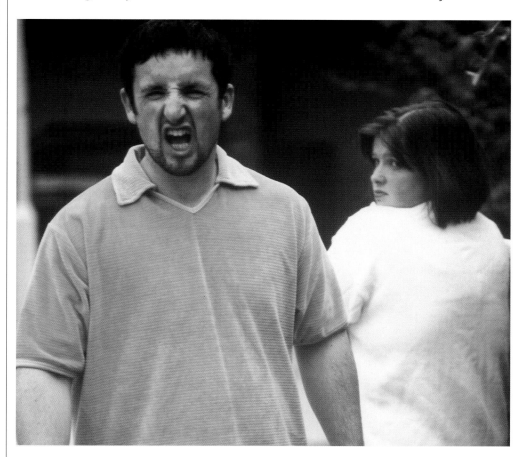

▲ *The sufferer from the rare condition called Tourette's syndrome is subject to involuntary grimaces and tics and, in more extreme cases, to episodes of barking, grunting, and obscene language.*

body are upset. In kidney or liver disease, muscle twitching may eventually become quite pronounced (see Kidneys and Kidney Diseases; Liver and Liver Disease).

Tics

Most tics are simply coordinated twitches that occur in groups of muscles, usually in the face and especially around the eyes. Basically, a tic differs from a twitch in that it is a repeated, coordinated, but purposeless twitch that often occurs in bursts. A tic is common in children between the ages of five and ten, and normally lasts for only a week or two. Usually, the tic causes only parental anxiety or teasing from other children. If, however, the child starts to become worried about it, that worrying can cause the tic to get worse.

The most common types of tic involve muscles around the eyes and mouth. The tic takes the form of a grimace or frown that transiently distorts the face and quickly disappears. The same pattern of movement, or expression, is repeated many times, often more frequently in stressful situations. Most people with tics have just one repetitive movement; however, occasionally people suffer from multiple tics, which may have completely different patterns.

Gilles de la Tourette's syndrome

On rare occasions, multiple tics may develop into the more serious Tourette's syndrome, named after the doctor who first described it, Gilles de la Tourette. It is not common, although it probably also occurs in a mild form that is often not diagnosed. It usually starts in the teens with the development of multiple tics and the appearance of odd grunts and shouts. The person's intelligence is usually normal, but the full-blown syndrome can give the sufferer a very strange appearance, and the multiple tics can often be severely disabling when they occur.

What causes tics?

The reason why some people develop persistent tics is not yet known. Although many psychological theories have been advanced to explain these abnormalities in terms of anxiety and stress, few have been accepted. It is believed that there is probably some electrical problem in the movement control centers of the brain, particularly those of the face, which have to control a large range of very sensitive muscle groups. There never appears to be any damage to these areas and a tic is never a symptom of a serious disease, so any abnormality in these control centers is probably only a temporary disturbance that eventually rights itself. When a tic becomes permanent or prolonged it is thought that the movement becomes an ingrained habit.

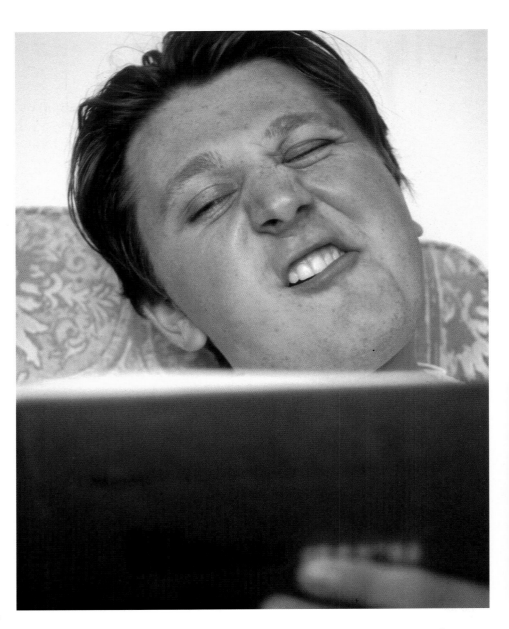

▲ *Facial tics can be distressing, but are momentary. However, severe twitching can be a symptom of liver or kidney disease.*

Myoclonus

Myoclonus is a sudden, large-scale twitch that we all sometimes get, especially when about to go to sleep. Severe persistent myoclonus can indicate brain degeneration, although this is rare and occurs with other signs of serious brain disease (see Brain; Brain Damage and Disease).

Treatment

In most cases no treatment, other than an explanation and reassurance, is needed for those who have a twitch or tic. When someone suffers from multiple tics, these may need to be suppressed, and there are several drugs that can help.

Myoclonus can usually be controlled, because drugs that are used for epilepsy seem to be effective (see Epilepsy).

See also: **Anxiety; Fatigue**

Typhoid and paratyphoid

Typhoid is still one of the most serious infectious fevers, but antibiotics and modern sanitation have gone a long way toward controlling it. Paratyphoid, as the name suggests, is a similar but less severe illness.

The serious infectious fevers typhus and typhoid have been recognized for centuries, but until the middle of the last century no distinction was made between them and they were both called typhus (see Typhus). In reality, the two diseases are quite distinct in their effects. Although typhoid, which affects the intestines in particular, was gradually recognized as a separate disease, its association with typhus remained, since the name "typhoid" simply means typhus-like. Paratyphoid is a disease very like typhoid but is considerably less severe.

Causes

Typhoid is caused by one of the salmonella organisms (see Salmonella), which are spread by contaminated food and water and give rise to food poisoning. *Salmonella typhi* (the typhoid organism) has developed to cause a generalized illness only in humans. There are three different

Questions and Answers

I have heard that typhoid is worse if you have gallstones. Is this true?

No. If you have gallstones you are more likely to become a carrier of the disease. The organism seems to settle in the gallbladder, and the presence of stones in the gallbladder makes this easier.

Can children catch typhoid?

Yes. However, the illness in children can be difficult for a doctor to recognize. The disease usually lasts for a shorter period and may seem to be primarily a respiratory illness.

Is typhoid treated with antibiotics?

Yes. Chloramphenicol was the main treatment for years but has been replaced by ciprofloxacin, which is highly effective. Typhoid can still be fatal but usually the illness responds well to treatment, and the fever settles after about five days rather than three weeks. Chloramphenicol had the serious disadvantage that in a very few patients it suppressed the bone marrow, so that blood cells were no longer produced. This was a fatal condition, but the risk that it will happen is much smaller than the risk of dying from untreated typhoid. Amoxicillin and co-trimoxazole are still used but the quinolone antibiotics such as ciprofloxacin are now preferred.

Can you catch typhoid from corned beef?

There was an outbreak in Scotland in 1964; contaminated water was sucked into a can of corned beef during the cooling period after the canning process. This was indirectly a waterborne infection; water contaminated with sewage is a common cause of typhoid outbreaks. However, canned foods are usually safe.

TYPHOID IN THE SMALL INTESTINE

▼ *A serious complication of typhoid occurs in the small intestine; the organism infects lymphatic tissue called Peyer's patches. They become inflamed and may ulcerate, causing perforation of the intestinal wall (insets).*

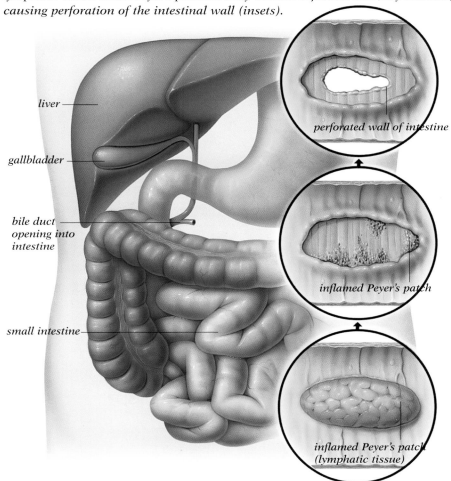

liver

gallbladder

bile duct opening into intestine

small intestine

perforated wall of intestine

inflamed Peyer's patch

inflamed Peyer's patch (lymphatic tissue)

Questions and Answers

In Greece last summer, I had the most dreadful bout of diarrhea. Could it have been typhoid?

No, that is most unlikely. Typhoid is a generalized disease affecting the whole body. If you do get diarrhea, it comes on late in the illness, after about two weeks. It is possible that the illness you had was caused by one of the salmonella organisms (as typhoid is), since these cause acute gastroenteritis. Paratyphoid can give you an illness similar to typhoid, but sometimes it just causes gastroenteritis.

Is it possible to catch typhoid from animals?

No. Typhoid seems to be an exclusively human disease, with one exception: fruit-eating bats in Madagascar. If you catch the disease, therefore, you must have caught it from someone else, via fecal contamination of food or water. It is unusual for typhoid to spread directly from person to person. On the other hand, paratyphoid seems to be less specialized and it can attack other animals. There is at least one outbreak on record in which cattle were the source of the infection.

I have heard the term "typhoid carrier," but what exactly does it mean?

Typhoid carriers are the main source of the infection. Once someone has been infected, and has recovered from the acute stage of the illness, the typhoid organisms may settle in the body and be excreted in the feces or urine without causing any serious symptoms. It is quite normal for people who have had the disease to excrete the organisms for about three months, but if this continues then they are called carriers. It is unusual for anyone under the age of 20 to become a carrier. The state of being a carrier is most likely to occur in middle-aged women. There are known cases of people carrying the organism for 50 years or possibly even longer.

Effects of typhoid on the body

ORGAN/SYSTEM	EFFECTS
Blood	Typhoid spreads into the bloodstream immediately after infection
Intestine	Organisms spread from the blood back into the wall of the intestine and may cause ulcers and bleeding, or lead to rupture of the intestinal wall
Skin	The typical typhoid rash takes the form of a few rose-red spots
Gallbladder	Typhoid is particularly likely to infect the gallbladder, which is the site of infection in carriers
Kidneys	The kidneys are also infected, and are another possible site of infection in carriers, who then pass infected urine
Lungs	A cough is common in the early stages, and pneumonia may occur; lung problems are common in children
Heart	The heart is involved in 5 to 10 percent of cases. This can lead to heart failure and can certainly be a cause of death.
Nervous system and psychiatric symptoms	The disease starts with a headache and patients become dull and confused. During the second week they become totally withdrawn until they are effectively in a coma—the "coma vigil." Sometimes there is an initial episode of severe psychiatric disturbance, and there can also be cases of meningitis, though these are rare.
Bones and joints	Abscesses can form under the periosteum (lining membrane) of bones after the acute stage of the disease. Joints can also be affected.

types of paratyphoid caused by the organisms *Salmonella paratyphi* A, B, and C. In the West, paratyphoid B is the only one of any real importance.

How infection is spread

Salmonella typhi survives so successfully because some infected people continue to pass the organism in their feces, yet remain quite fit and free of symptoms. Such people are called carriers, and are ideal hosts for the organism, which tends to settle in the gallbladder and remain there for years while new organisms are excreted into the intestine via the bile duct.

In the past, food and water became readily contaminated with human feces, and this enabled typhoid to become very widespread. It is perhaps this disease more than any other that owes its successful eradication in the 20th-century West to modern techniques of hygiene and sanitation (see Public Health).

Another reason the organism is so well adapted to infect humans is that it survives well in fresh water and many serious epidemics have been waterborne. Organisms can, however, survive for any length of time in water only if there is decaying organic matter present for them to feed on. If water is stored in a clean reservoir the number of organisms will be reduced.

Salmonella typhi do not survive well in seawater, so there is little risk of catching typhoid by sunbathing on a polluted beach. It is, however, undesirable for coastal towns to discharge raw sewage into the sea. Shellfish filter gallons of water to extract their food, and sewage may certainly contaminate seafood.

Dairy produce is a fairly common source of infection, since it provides an excellent medium in which the bacteria can grow. Infected milk almost always occurs through a human carrier, and less often by contamination with sewage. Typhoid can of course be spread by any food, although the organism is destroyed by thorough cooking (see Food Poisoning). A carrier who works with food is especially dangerous, since there is a very high risk of fecal contamination of the hands. The most famous carrier of all was an American cook who was known as Typhoid Mary.

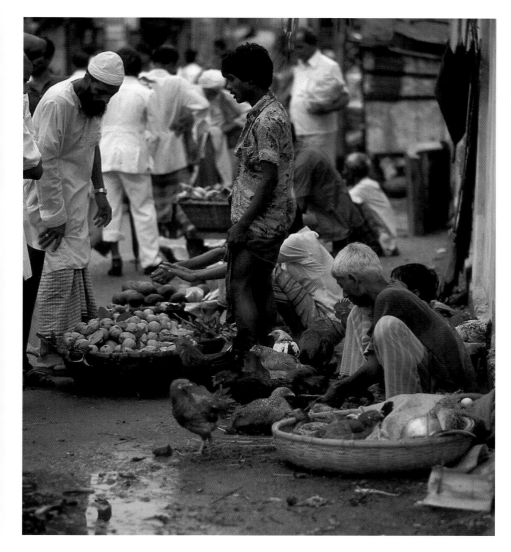

▲ *The typhoid organism is carried in human feces, which can contaminate food and water in unsanitary surroundings, like this street market in Bangladesh. Far fewer epidemics occur in the West, where there are higher standards of hygiene.*

Symptoms

Typhoid has an incubation period of between 10 and 14 days. It begins as a flulike illness with symptoms of a headache, muscle pains, and abdominal discomfort. Initially, constipation (see Constipation) is common, and diarrhea (see Diarrhea) occurs occasionally.

The fever rises slowly over the course of a week or so (see Fevers; Temperature). The temperature is always raised in the evening, but usually falls slightly by the following morning until it finally reaches 104°F (40°C) by the end of a week.

By the end of the first week, the patient obviously has a serious disease and is in a poor general condition with a severe headache. At this stage, chest symptoms are very common and sometimes pneumonia develops (see Pneumonia). The abdomen is distended, and two of the most significant symptoms will be present: the spleen can be felt in the top left-hand corner of the abdomen, and a few pale pink patches appear on the skin.

The organism can be grown in cultures of the blood during the course of the first week, and this is often how the diagnosis is made. The organisms are so widespread after about a week that they can also be grown in culture from a specimen of skin containing a rose-red spot.

During the second week of the disease, patients become progressively sicker, with particular deterioration in their mental function and withdrawal from what is happening around them.

Throughout the first two weeks the organism is passing from the blood into various organs of the body, but it is in the intestines that serious complications can occur. At intervals down the length of the small intestine there are collections of lymphatic tissue called Peyer's patches. Typhoid tends to infect these in particular, and their surfaces may ulcerate, causing severe intestinal bleeding.

By the third week an untreated patient is extremely ill, with a swollen abdomen and a stupor that almost amounts to a coma. Diarrhea occurs at this stage, since the intestines become involved, but more serious than this is the risk that the walls of the intestine might perforate, particularly around the Peyer's patches.

If this does not happen, then the fever begins to settle after three or four weeks, although there is a high risk of a possibly serious relapse.

The carrier state

It is normal for the salmonella organisms to persist in the patient's stools for as long as three months, and they have to be investigated regularly for this reason. Patients who are still excreting the organisms have to continue to take special precautions. In some patients, the carrier state persists, although this is uncommon in anyone who is below the age of 20. Middle-aged women are, in fact, most likely to become carriers; the ratio of male to female carriers is roughly one to three.

Anyone who has recovered from typhoid should always be extremely careful about hygiene. Washing the hands after using the toilet is a basic precaution that will prevent the spread of this debilitating disease (see Hygiene).

Treatment

A diagnosis is made either by developing a culture of the typhoid bacteria from specimens of the patient's blood, feces, or urine (see Laboratory Tests; Specimens), or by means of a blood test that reveals the presence of antibodies to the bacteria.

The antibiotic chloramphenicol made a great difference to the treatment of the disease, and once it was started the illness usually settled within about five days. However, the drug could cause fatal depression of the bone marrow so that no blood cells were produced. Although this is a rare condition, it meant that this antibiotic had to be reserved for potentially fatal illnesses such as typhoid. A later drug, ciprofloxacin, is now much more frequently

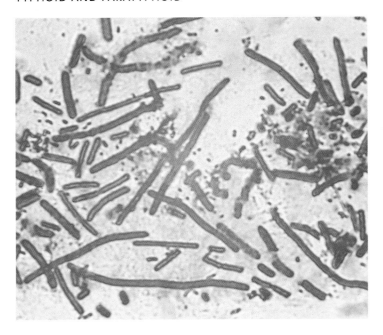

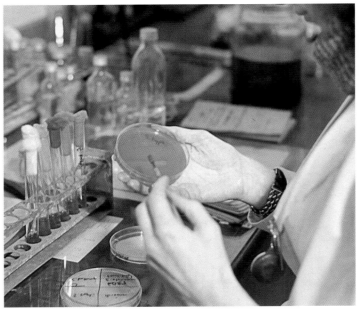

▲ *The typhoid bacillus and the less virulent paratyphoid strain are two of a large group of organisms called salmonellae. Typhoid and paratyphoid mainly infect humans and have a tendency to remain in the body in a carrier state.*

▲ *A specimen is placed on a culture plate; then it will be examined under a microscope. The organisms may persist in the patient's stools for as long as three months after the disease has run its course, and in rare cases for much longer.*

used and is at least as effective as chloramphenicol, but without the same side effects (see Side Effects).

Occasionally, in extremely severe cases, patients may require supplementary treatment with corticosteroid drugs, which reduce inflammation in the intestine. Surgery may also be required if the patient suffers widespread peritonitis or severe bleeding.

▼ *Diagnosis of the disease can be made in the first week if a culture of the blood is taken and colonies of the bacillus are found. Classic symptoms of the disease are a distended abdomen and the appearance of rose-red spots—pale pink patches on the skin. When someone is suspected of having typhoid or of being a carrier, his or her feces are investigated since these may be contaminated with the organism.*

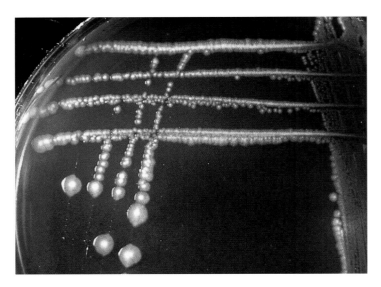

Prevention

Typhoid is mainly prevented by the control of sewage disposal and the provision of clean water supplies, as well as rigorous hygiene.

A useful and reliable vaccine against typhoid is available, and anyone who is traveling to a country where the standards of hygiene are low would be advised to get the vaccine. It is called TAB, meaning "typhoid and paratyphoid A and B," and is about 70 percent effective at preventing typhoid if someone is infected. A booster is needed after about three years.

Paratyphoid

Paratyphoid closely resembles typhoid in many respects, but it is caused by a different bacterium called *Salmonella paratyphi*. Carriers of paratyphoid exist, but are not responsible for all outbreaks of the disease. The incubation period is shorter, and paratyphoid is not as infectious as typhoid. Therefore, someone who has contracted the organism will not necessarily get the disease. Paratyphoid causes symptoms resembling both typhoid and salmonella poisoning. There is an acute phase of gastroenteritis (see Gastroenteritis) but no generalized disease develops, and only in very rare cases does paratyphoid prove to be fatal.

Outlook

Since only eight cases of typhoid were reported to CDC in 2002, it seems that typhoid may be a problem of the past in the West; but elsewhere in the world, usually wherever sanitation is poor, typhoid epidemics are, tragically, a regular feature of life. The vast majority of the cases that occur in the United States are contracted abroad. Prompt diagnosis and treatment of the disease ensure a good outlook for patients with typhoid.

See also: **Bacteria; Spleen**

Typhus

Questions and Answers

Typhus is a disease that waits in the wings to strike at humanity when social breakdown occurs. If normal hygiene measures deteriorate, this louse-borne illness spreads rapidly from person to person.

There are actually a number of typhus illnesses, all caused by the same type of organisms—the rickettsiae. Rickettsiae are spread from human to human by bloodsucking insects.

The most serious form of typhus is called epidemic typhus, and it is common in the social breakdown that can follow such disasters as war, famine, floods, and earthquakes. A less serious disease is murine typhus. This is basically a disease of rats, and it spreads to humans via the rat flea. Finally, there is a disease of the east called scrub typhus or tsutsugamushi fever.

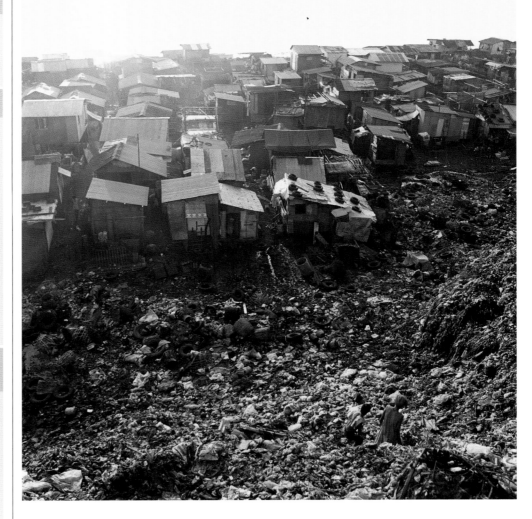

▲ *Overcrowded, desperately unhygienic living conditions are perfect breeding grounds for epidemic typhus. The disease is mainly found in Africa and South America.*

Questions and Answers

My father died of typhus when he liberated a concentration camp at the end of World War II. Why was typhus common in the camps?

Typhus is found when normal social organization has broken down. The disease depends upon the louse for transmission from human to human, and this occurs only if hygiene is poor. Also, typhus is a disease that thrives in cold conditions, such as the concentration camps in Europe.

Is it true that typhus can cause gangrene?

Yes. In severe cases of the disease there may be gangrene of the extremities, such as the fingers and toes, ears, and genitals.

How do lice spread typhus?

When a louse bites in order to eat blood, it defecates at the same time, and louse feces contain the infection. When the bite is scratched, the infection contained in the feces is rubbed into the skin and the disease starts. The infection seems to be able to survive in louse feces for a long time, so the dust from the clothes of a person who is louse-ridden can be very infective. The disease also causes the death of infected lice, and their corpses also provide a source of infection in dust from clothing.

Does epidemic typhus infect any animals other than man?

It is believe to infect only one other species, the flying squirrel of North America. However, murine typhus seems to be primarily a disease of rats and it occurs where rats are common, for example in seaports. Murine typhus causes a similar but less severe disease in man; but it can still be serious.

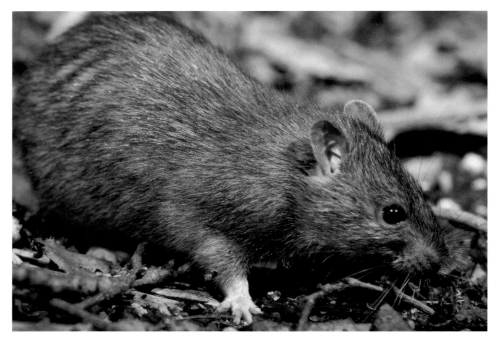

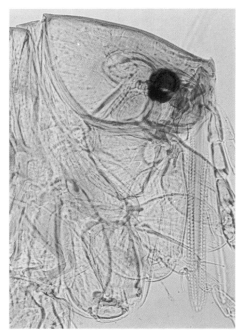

▲ *The black rat carries a flea that is responsible for a rare disease, murine typhus, also called endemic typhus.*

▲ *Rickettsiae are the organisms that cause typhus; they are carried by bloodsucking insects such as chiggers (above right), which cause scrub typhus.*

Causes of epidemic typhus

The organism of epidemic typhus is called *Rickettsia prowazekii* and the infection is transmitted from human to human by infected body lice; it cannot be caught directly from another human.

Epidemic typhus is rare in most developed countries and occurs in communities where lice infestations are frequent and housing conditions are overcrowded and unhygienic. For example, it is typically seen in refugee camps and prisoner populations, especially during wars, famines, and natural disasters, where damage has been inflicted on housing and water supplies.

A louse becomes infected by sucking an infected person's blood, but another human has to be very close for the louse to transfer.

Once a louse is infected, the rickettsiae grow in its intestine and are passed out in the feces. Invariably, the louse defecates as it eats, leading to transfer of infection, since the human host will scratch the irritating bite and rub the feces into the wound. Rickettsiae live for a long time in louse feces, and the dust from infected clothing can be very infectious.

Symptoms and diagnosis

The incubation period for epidemic typhus is about 10 days to three weeks. The disease causes flulike symptoms: it starts very suddenly with a high fever; the patient feels sick, with muscular aches and pains; and there is also a headache.

A rash appears after three or four days: it begins gradually and can simply be mistaken for the flush of a fever. However, it becomes more widespread and consists of small red flat spots. After about a week or so it gets darker, and the spots may start to look more blotchy and rather like little bruises. The most serious stage of the disease occurs as the rash gets more obvious (see Rashes). Patients sink into a stupor and, although they are awake, it is often impossible to communicate with them. Delirium and coma can then occur. At this point the deterioration can be very alarming: the

kidneys start to fail; a cough develops; and the rash may actually progress to gangrene in the fingers, toes, and genitals. Dangerous complications, such as pneumonia, often occur. In untreated infections, somewhere between 20 and 50 percent of patients will die at this stage. Those who are going to recover lose their fever in the third week and the brain starts working normally very quickly. However, they will need a very long period of convalescence. Although diagnosis can usually be made from the symptoms, sometimes a blood test is done to confirm the diagnosis. However, if typhus is suspected, it is usual for a doctor to initiate treatment on the basis of clinical observation rather than waiting for the results of confirmatory tests from a laboratory.

Treatment

The condition responds to treatment with certain antibiotics and supportive care. The drugs most likely to be successful in controlling the infection are tetracycline and chloramphenicol. Often, however, in the squalid circumstances where lice spread, antibiotics are not readily available (see Antibiotics). If no treatment is given, the disease can stay in the body in a dormant state and can be reactivated years later.

Murine and scrub typhus

Murine typhus is less severe than epidemic typhus and the death rate without treatment is probably about 2 percent. Murine typhus is a disease that is found where humans are in quite close contact with rats. For example, it is often endemic in rat-infested areas such as ports and food stores.

Most people who get scrub typhus first notice a black scab at the site of the bite, and a characteristic feature of scrub typhus is that 60 percent of infected people develop a hard scar at the site of the infecting bite within about five days. This scar is called an eschar. The

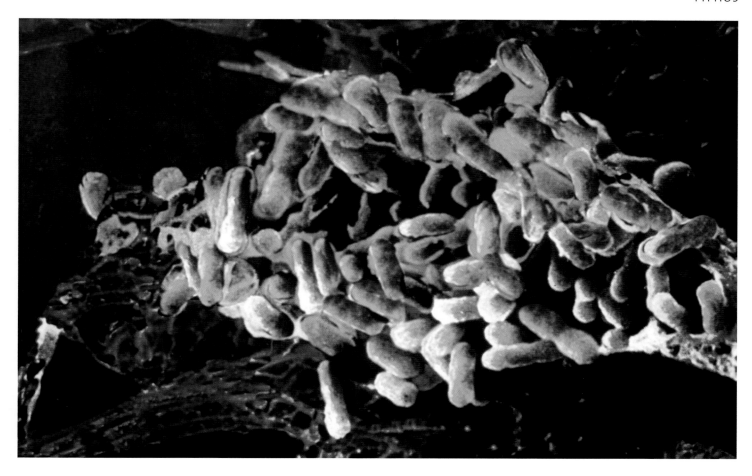

▲ *A colorized scanning electron micrograph of* Rickettsia prowazekii, *which is spread by insects and causes epidemic typhus.*

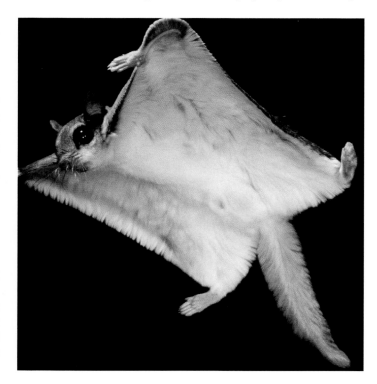

▲ *Epidemic typhus is believed to infect only one animal: the flying squirrel.*

disease then goes on in a way that is very similar to epidemic typhus. The illness exists in a large number of animals and is spread by a bloodsucking mite or chigger. As the name suggests, scrub typhus is a disease that occurs in scrubland when the free-living chiggers leave the scrubby undergrowth to bite and infect.

Prevention

Vaccine against typhus does exist, and it provides good protection. It is also possible to take tetracycline when traveling in an infected area (see Vaccinations). Travelers are unlikely to contract typhus unless they are in close contact with people who have lice. However, health workers are at risk of lice-borne infections because they may become infected through inhaling or being inoculated with infectious louse feces.

The single most important means of prevention is to control the fleas and lice that carry the disease. In the case of epidemic typhus this is not too difficult, since the louse is fairly easy to deal with. In areas with murine typhus authorities can only attempt an eradication program to destroy rats, but this is a major undertaking.

The most serious control problem is that of scrub typhus, a disease found in rural areas. There are many small animals in which the disease can survive; in fact, humans are probably an unusual host to this infection.

See also: Bites and stings; Fevers; Tetracyclines; Vaccinations

INDEX